W9-BFN-110

Cooking for
DIABETICS

Cooking for
DIABETICS

Kitty E. Maynard, R.N.
Lucian Maynard, R.N.
Theodore G. Duncan, M.D.

Julia M. Pitkin, Editor

Rutledge Hill Press
Nashville, Tennessee

Dedicated to

the loyal patrons of Miss Kitty's Pie in the Sky
Specialty Bakery
— without you we would not have ventured so far —
and to those we have not yet served

Copyright © 1989 Lucian Maynard, Kitty E. Maynard, and Theodore G.
Duncan

Published in Nashville, Tennessee by Rutledge Hill Press, Inc.
211 Seventh Avenue North, Nashville, Tennessee 37219

The exchange lists are the basis of a meal planning system designed by a
committee of the American Diabetes Association and The American Dietetic
Association. While designed primarily for people with diabetes and others
who must follow special diets, the exchange lists are based on principles of
good nutrition that apply to everyone. © 1986 American Diabetes
Association, The American Dietetic Association.

Nutritional analysis: Nancy Casillas, M.S., R.D.
Typography: Bailey Typography
Design: Harriette Bateman

Library of Congress Cataloging-in-Publication Data

Maynard, Kitty E., 1955-
    Cooking for diabetics.

    Includes index.
    1. Diabetes — Diet therapy — Recipes.   I. Maynard,
Lucian, 1952-   II. Duncan, Theodore G.
III. Title
RC662.M38   1989   641.5'6314   88-32374
ISBN 1-55853-000-2

Printed in the United States of America
            12 13 14 15 — 99 98 97

Introduction

Nearly fourteen years ago I enrolled in nursing school. One year later, Lucian followed. Ours was one of those old-fashioned three-year schools: heavy on clinical experience in addition to a tough academic program. We were drilled and redrilled daily on care and teaching. We were taught to instruct our patients on how to return to their daily routines without a loss of autonomy. At the time learning all those teaching and instructional plans seemed like busywork.

Ten years of working in hospital settings in Intensive Care Units of all types — medical, surgical, neurological, cardiac, and open heart recovery — taught us how important our instructional teaching had been, but we noticed that the diabetic presented a special challenge. Patients with diabetes, whether newly diagnosed or veterans, needed extra teaching to adjust their lifestyles to include the preparation of foods.

Unfortunately, this teaching was done poorly in the hospital setting. Instead of practical lessons in food preparation, diabetics were given literature and exchange lists and sent on their way. In contrast, stroke patients received considerable practical experience in working within a set-up kitchen and a home setting in their rehabilitation. Who would work with diabetics on those meals that suddenly had become so terribly important?

A lot can be said for the dietician's role in food preparation within the hospital. Today hospitals give a greater emphasis on adjusting and using recipes for diabetics. Thankfully, organizations such as the American Diabetes Association have made hospitals aware of diabetics' needs. Even so, as nurses we continued to hear our patients tell us that they needed better diabetic foods. After all, preparing diabetic meals never comes easy; and fear of the unknown — the thought that you may make an error that will cause a reaction — is very common.

Christmas of 1981 was a turning point for us, for we made a decision that has affected our lives far beyond what we could have imagined at the time. Lucian and I were working at the hospital on Christmas day, and three consecutive patients who were admitted had extremely high blood sugars. When histories were taken from their families, we found that all three patients had been depressed and frustrated over the lack of tasty foods for them. So they ate what they wanted, not what they should.

On our way home that evening, we talked about the problems these three patients were experiencing. We didn't stop once we arrived at home, and for the next year we continued to hear frustration from diabetic patients about their food problems. As we continued to listen to our patients, we realized this problem was not unique to diabetics. Those with cholesterol or sodium restricted diets were experiencing the same frustrations, as were those with multiple food allergies.

In 1987 Lucian and I finally struck out on our own by starting a specialty bakery, although we had planned and experimented for a full year before opening our doors. In that time we created good tasting, nutritious recipes of our own. We worked closely with the American Diabetic Association, the American Heart Association, and a few weight reduction programs in developing our foods.

Our experience at the bakery has been exciting and rewarding, especially the satisfaction of watching our customers' pleasure in finding new avenues for eating right and enjoying food once again. We have taken great pride and joy in watching the faces of children who now — for the first time ever — are able to enjoy the simple pleasure of eating their own birthday cake. That may not seem like much to some, but it means a great deal to us.

Our bakery has allowed us to carry our nursing experience into new areas. We do not see owning a bakery as a new career, but as an extension of our commitment to nursing. In our bakery we are able to spend time with our customers to explain how the exchange lists work and how they should prepare meals in their own homes. They bring us recipes that have given them trouble, and we help them adjust the ingredients to their dietary needs. We give family members helpful hints on how to care for diabetics in their families, and we also refer them to their physicians or dieticians if they need additional help. Our motto is, "Ask us your questions. If we can't answer them, we'll find someone who can."

Cooking for Diabetics is written in answer to repeated requests from our friends and customers. Hardly a day has gone by in which we have not had numerous requests for recipes that could be used in their homes. After *The American Country Inn and Bed & Breakfast Cookbook* was published in August of 1987, they began to ask for a book on diabetic cooking, too. This book, then, is our answer to their requests.

Thanks guys. You all are the best!

— Kitty and Lucian Maynard

Contents

INTRODUCTION, *v*

STRAIGHT TALK ABOUT DIET AND
DIABETES, *1*

PRACTICAL TIPS FOR LIVING WITH
DIABETES, *9*

A GUIDE TO MEAL PLANNING, *17*

APPETIZERS, *37*

BEVERAGES, *49*

SALADS, *69*

SOUPS, *91*

BREADS, *113*

ENTREES, *131*

VEGETABLES AND RICE, *169*

DESSERTS, *189*

MISCELLANEOUS, *213*

INDEXES, *219*

Acknowledgments

We are pleased to acknowledge the following organizations for providing photographs for the color inserts: Evans Food Group, Pacific Kitchens Division (Golden Apple Wheat Bread, Skillet Apple Potato Salad, Stuffed Chicken Breasts); Florida Department of Natural Resources, Bureau of Seafood Marketing (Ale-Poached Fish with Pimiento Sauce, Lettuce Baked Lobster Tails, Rock Shrimp and Oyster Manquechou); Hershey Foods Corporation (Gazpacho Salad, Manicotti with Eggplant-Tomato Relish, Manicotti with Ratatouille Sauce, Mostaccioli al Forno, Pasta Salad, Savory Jumbo Shells); International Apple Institute (Spicy Applesauce); Kitchens of Sara Lee (Light and Easy Pound Cake); National Fisheries Institute (Crab Soup, Shrimp and Oyster Gumbo, Tuna Chowder); National Livestock and Meat Board (Holiday Beef Steaks with Vegetable Sauté and Hot Mustard Sauce, Microwave Beef Roast and Fennel Parmesan, Oriental Beef Kabobs, Poached Beef Tenderloin with Steamed Vegetables).

Cooking for
DIABETICS

Straight Talk about Diet and Diabetes

*D*iets of one kind or another are on every-one's lips these days. And diet plans — good and bad — have multiplied like rabbits. There are diets extolling high fiber, fish and rice, rice and vegetables, high fat, low fat, high protein, low protein — the list is endless. Many such diets are nutritionally sound, others are not; but their very number means that we are at last becoming conscious of the vital importance of diet in our lives. Nevertheless, many persons do not really understand the essence of a good diet or what it contributes to health.

Both diet and exercise are essential to good health. We have only to look at the eating and exercise patterns of various populations over the past few decades to learn that decreased exercise combined with an over-abundance of foods — especially those rich in saturated fats and cholesterol — increases the rate of new onset of diabetes and heart disease. Fortunately, the reverse is also true. In World War II, for instance, increased activity and reduced availability of food decreased the number of new cases of diabetes by 40 percent in both Germany and En-gland. The rate remained low during the war and did not rise again until the Marshall Plan provided ample food for Germany and other parts of Europe. While humanitarian in its intent, the supply of food was nevertheless followed by a stunning increase in new cases of diabetes. Similarly, before 1945 diabetes was essentially nonexistent among Eskimos and American Indians. But once these populations adopted our "civilized" eating and activity patterns, the incidence of diabetes also increased markedly.

There is no longer any doubt about the correlation between what we eat, how active we are, and the incidence of specific diseases. In the past ten years, since we learned that obesity, saturated fats, and cholesterol are risk factors for heart disease, many Americans have been working to decrease the risk by eating fewer eggs and high fat dairy products (such as ice cream and whipped cream) and less fatty meats, turning instead to fish, chicken, turkey, and low fat dairy products. Since these diets are being combined with increased exercise, new cases of heart disease have decreased 40 percent in this same decade, a decrease that can be attributed directly to changes in dietary and exercise patterns.

Disease rarely concerns any of us when we are young; unfortunately, as we now know, we cannot afford to postpone safe dietary and activity habits to middle age. Medical research has clearly demonstrated that early signs of coronary disease can be found in a majority of Americans between the ages of eighteen and twenty-five. By instituting the proper diet earlier in life, we can eliminate such changes. By the time we reach age twenty, we have each eaten more than twenty-four tons of food. Clearly, it is important that it be the right kind of food.

Healthy persons can readily metabolize most nutrient components of their diet, using what they need for energy and the maintenance of body structure. But if we take in too many calories, we become fat; if we don't eat enough, we develop malnutrition. Even in obesity the body can cope with most of the nutritional components of the diet, but cholesterol is different. This compound is not eliminated easily, and excess amounts are apt to be stored in the walls of the arteries in general and in the coronary blood vessels in particular. Unchecked, this will ultimately lead to coronary artery disease. More diabetics have high cholesterol and heart disease than do normal persons. Thus, paying particular attention to the fat and cholesterol components of the diet can help eliminate or postpone coronary artery disease.

What impact does diet have on diabetes?

To answer that question, let's look at what diabetes is and how it affects the body. Diabetes is a chronic, systemic disease characterized by disorders of metabolism that elevate blood sugar and, sometimes, blood lipids. There are two well-recognized types: Type I, usually called juvenile-onset diabetes, and Type II, usually called maturity-onset diabetes. Over eleven million Americans have diabetes; ninety percent of them (most of whom are obese) have Type II, while ten percent have "brittle" Type I juvenile diabetes and require insulin treatment.

Type I diabetes usually occurs before puberty. The onset is abrupt, and the patient is usually undernourished. Because of the elevated blood sugar, the patient initially urinates frequently, is very thirsty, and has a ravenous appetite. Once insulin therapy brings the blood sugar under control, these symptoms disappear. Blood sugar fluctuates widely in response to small changes in insulin dosage, exercise, and stress; thus, control of the Type I diabetic is more difficult. Many Type I diabetic patients follow the American Diabetes Association diet and eat three meals and prescribed snacks on time to help maintain control and prevent low blood sugars (more about this later). Insulin is the only drug that can control this type of diabetes.

Type II, or maturity-onset diabetes, commonly develops after age thirty-five. The onset is gradual. It is commonly found in obese persons with a positive family history for the disease. Often, patients have no symptoms and may unknowingly have elevated blood sugars for years before symptoms begin. Once the patient begins treatment, blood sugar fluctuations are less marked; often the diabetes can be controlled by diet alone or, if not, by the use of a pill, an oral hypoglycemic agent. If diet is correctly used, hypoglycemic therapy may not be necessary. In fact, we believe that as many as eighty-five percent of Type II diabetic patients would require no medication if they reduced their weight to normal. Unhappily, not many persons are motivated highly enough to achieve this task and tend to succumb to such temptations as butter, chocolate, and other sweets. However, when an ideal diabetic diet is presented through tantalizing diets and menus, such as those illustrated in this book, we have hope that the success rate will increase.

How do we design a diabetic diet?

The first time you look at it, the so-called "diabetic diet" may appear rather complex, especially if you have just learned that you have diabetes or have not dieted before. Yet, on examination the diet proves not only understandable, but simple to follow. Like any other nutritionally balanced diet, the diabetic diet fulfills certain criteria. Total daily caloric needs are estimated to provide enough calories for energy and tissue building — usually by either a physician or a dietitian. The diet-maker also calculates the necessary proportions of fat, carbohydrate, protein, essential vitamins, and minerals. Some diabetics, especially those taking insulin, also need help with the appropriate timing of regular meals and snacks to prevent low blood sugar reactions.

As noted earlier, diabetic patients have some special problems. About fifty percent have hypertension — high blood pressure — their diets should include sodium restriction. If you have hypertension, you should ingest no more than 2 grams of sodium daily; to reach this goal, you must eliminate salt from both the kitchen and the dining room. One way to do this is to throw away the salt shakers; another is to fill them with sodium-free spices instead. Similarly, patients with elevated cholesterol levels must stick to a low saturated fat/low-cholesterol diet. Often, diet adjustments alone can lower cholesterol values to within normal limits, thus decreasing the coronary risk factor. Sometimes kidney problems complicate diabetes. Recent studies show that if we limit dietary protein to about forty grams per day, we can reduce the work of the kidneys and, perhaps, slow the progression of renal disease.

How do we calculate ideal weight and caloric intake?

Diet is as essential to the treatment of diabetes as insulin, oral hypoglycemic medications, and exercise. As a diabetic, you must plan your diet to maintain ideal weight, eating the proper proportions of fat, carbohydrate, protein, and other nutrients essential to good health. First and foremost, consider food as a source of energy needed by your body for physical and mental activity and the maintenance of tissues and structures. If you eat more calories than you need, your body will store them as fat and you will gain weight. If you don't eat enough, you will become malnourished and lose weight. The total number of calories each person needs varies with body build, gender, and activity.

An adult woman should weigh one hundred pounds for the first five feet in height and an additional five pounds for each inch over five feet. An adult man is allotted 106 pounds for the first five feet and six pounds for each additional inch. If the person has a small frame, subtract 10 percent; and if the person has a large frame, add 10 percent. For example, a woman with a medium frame, height 5'4", has an ideal weight of 120 pounds (100 + 20 [5 lb. x 4"]). A six foot tall man with a large frame has an ideal weight of 196 pounds. (106 + 72 [6 lb. x 12"] = 178 pounds. + 10% [18 lbs] = 196 pounds).

To determine the number of daily calories needed to maintain ideal body weight, multiply the ideal weight by ten. If ideal body weight is 130 pounds, the basal number of calories needed every twenty-four hours is 1,300. This does not allow for activity: a woman with average activity should eat approximately thirty percent more calories to provide energy. Thus, her diet should contain about 1,700 calories. If ideal body weight is two hundred pounds, the ideal basal calories needed each day is two thousand. A man engaged in strenuous physical labor may need fifty percent more calories to allow for this exercise. Thus, his diet could be increased to approximately three to four thousand calories per day.

Obesity remains a particularly vexing and perplexing problem. Of the almost innumerable dietary methods and medications tried, very few have yielded meaningful results. In fact, a weight reduction program works only if the patient makes a real commitment to it, an "I will" commitment, not a weak "I'll try." A weight reduction diet should be designed to allow the patient to lose one or two pounds per week until the ideal weight is achieved. It may take a month or a year. Rapid weight loss and fad diets simply do not work, and they do not offer the patient time to learn the right way to eat. The slow reduction of weight over a period of time allows the patient's mind and body to adjust to the lower caloric intake.

Although there are a great many variables, eliminating one thousand calories per day allows you to lose about two pounds per week; if you cut only 500 calories per day from your diet, you will lose only one pound each week — but think about it — one pound per week is 52 pounds per year! An excess weight of one hundred pounds represents 350,000 calories. If you eliminate one thousand calories from the diet that normally maintains ideal weight, it will take approximately 350 days to reach your ideal weight.

How can you get the most from the exchange lists?

Exchange lists for meal planning prepared by the American Diabetes Association, the American Dietetic Association, and the U.S. Public Health Service have provided an effective guide for the selection of mealtime and snack foods for over three decades.

Foods are divided into six basic groups including milk, vegetable, fruit, bread (carbohydrate), meat, and fat exchanges. Each food in a group contains the same number of calories as other foods in that specific list. In the fruit exchange list, for example, one medium-sized apple has sixty calories; so do twelve grapes, one small nectarine, or one-half cup of orange juice, and about three dozen others on the list. These can be used interchangeably to provide greater flexibility — and less monotony — when selecting fruit for dessert or a snack. The amount of food selected from exchange lists for each meal varies according to the total daily caloric requirement. The menu itself is selected from a daily menu guide that provides diets from 800 to 3,500 calories, which should be carefully and thoroughly explained, usually by a dietitian or diabetes nurse educator. Most foods are measured, not weighed. As with the fruit exchange, (sixty calories each), each exchange list is preceded by the number of calories provided in each serving in that list. Each item in the starch/bread exchange list is eighty calories, lean meat exchanges are fifty-five calories each and fatty meats are one hundred.

Once you gain experience using the exchange lists, you will find it quite easy to choose the right number of exchanges for each meal. The lists also indicate which foods contain excessive salt or have high fiber content. You will find this a most valuable and easy-to-understand dietary management system. Some patients, especially those needing insulin to control diabetes, must eat at regularly scheduled times and take between-meal snacks. Insulin lowers the blood sugar and if blood sugar becomes too low, hypoglycemia or insulin shock occurs. Long periods of fast — between meals and during the night — are potential danger times for hypoglycemia. Eating meals on time and adding between-meal and bedtime snacks help lessen the risk. In fact, the majority of diabetic control problems can be solved by adhering to the proper diet with proper meal times and snacks.

What does exercise contribute?

Exercise is an integral part of the treatment for diabetes. It reduces blood sugar by using up calories and enhances circulation throughout the blood vessels. It also improves muscle tone and helps reduce weight. Patients who participate in a continuing active exercise program maintain better blood sugar control, live longer, and have a better quality of life. An aerobic program that maintains a heart rate of about seventy-five to eighty percent of maximum, performed for thirty minutes at least three times per week, has been proven successful. A popular book, *The New Aerobic Way* by Dr. Kenneth Cooper, provides excellent, detailed exercise programs for achieving maximum benefits from the aerobic method.

Just as gasoline powers your car, glucose in the blood provides energy for the body; increased traveling or exercise uses more gasoline or glucose. When you exercise, you must compensate for the effect of exercise on blood sugar by increasing caloric intake. If you exercise more than average, take sugar orally to maintain blood sugar values above the hypoglycemic range. Have a glass of orange juice or cola, or candy before the exercise and an additional snack every hour during the exercise. *Do not wait until low blood sugar symptoms occur.* Increasing the sugar intake will provide you with a greater degree of safety and let you participate in all the physical activities you wish without the fear of experiencing low blood sugar reaction.

What about special dietary components?

Fiber The high fiber/high carbohydrate diet has generated a good deal of interest in recent years. Research has shown that a diet high in soluble fiber can help reduce the need for insulin or oral hypoglycemics and that some patients with non-insulin dependent diabetes can eliminate diabetes medication altogether through a program containing a high fiber diet, exercise, and weight loss. Fiber is not digested, but it absorbs water and encourages the passage of other foods through the digestive tract. It is found in fruits, vegetables, cereals, grains, and beans. There are two types of fiber. The *water soluble fiber* found in beans, oats, and fruits may help decrease blood cholesterol and help control blood sugar values. *Water insoluble fiber* provides bulk and, according to some studies, can decrease the risk of colon cancer. Because it is bulky and helps to curb the appetite, fiber also helps people lose weight. Research is ongoing, as the effect of high fiber foods on other nutrients in the diet is not yet clear. If you use fiber, add it to your diet gradually to allow the body to adjust. The current recommendations are from twenty to fifty grams per day.

Fruits with high soluble fiber content include blueberries, nectarines, pomegranates, raspberries, apples, apricots, figs, and prunes. Zucchini, cabbage, beans, peas, lentils, bran cereals, wheat germ, corn, and rye and pumpernickel breads also contain high amounts of fiber.

Cholesterol Patients with cholesterol values above 200 mg should follow an appropriate cholesterol-lowering diet to reduce this blood lipid. For every percentage point you are able to decrease your blood cholesterol value, you decrease your cardiac risk factor by two percent. As a population, Americans tend to eat large amounts of oils in foods and in whole milk and eggs, which cause excess cholesterol and fats to accumulate. Fats, particularly saturated fats, add to the problem of elevated cholesterol. Saturated fats are found chiefly in foods of animal origin, while unsaturated fats occur mainly in plants and fish. A low cholesterol/low fat diet includes fish, poultry without the skin, no fried foods, and limited use of eggs (three or less per week). Ask the advice of a dietitian to obtain a full explanation of how to use a cholesterol-lowering diet.

Alcohol There are many questions about alcoholic beverages in the diabetic diet. Should they be totally excluded? Are they safe? How do they influence control of blood sugar? In fact, the primary problem is calories — empty calories with no nutritional value. Hard liquor (whiskey, bourbon, rye, gin, brandy, rum) contains about 80 calories per ounce, one glass of beer has 80 to 150 calories, and a 3½ ounce glass of dry wine has 80 calories. If you are on a weight loss diet, you should exclude alcohol entirely, as it not only adds useless calories but decreases motivation. Obviously, patients having difficulty in controlling diabetes should attempt to "tighten up" all factors to improve this condition — including elimination of alcohol — until control has improved. Overall, it is best for a diabetic not to drink. If you do, do so sparingly. You might consider a glass of dry wine before dinner or a jigger of Scotch, preferably with soda or a non-caloric beverage.

The Sugars

The sugars come in many names and forms. Some sweeteners are acceptable under certain conditions, and as yet there are no established guidelines for their uses. The decision to employ these sweeteners is made on an individual basis. There are two categories of sweeteners — caloric and non-caloric. All caloric sugars provide 4 calories per gram or approximately 120 calories per ounce of weight. But there is a difference in the sweetness.

Sucrose Table sugar, as sucrose is more commonly known, is a combination of glucose and fructose that is extracted from sugar beets and cane. Light, dark, brown, and raw sugar are all sucrose and each conveys the same number of calories when eaten. Invert sugar commonly used by candy manufacturers and commercial bakers is made by processing sucrose so that it breaks down into free glucose and fructose. If ingested, glucose causes a rapid increase in blood sugar and should be avoided.

Fructose Many persons do not yet realize that fructose is a form of sugar and thus has calories that must be taken into consideration. Fructose is a very sweet form of sugar (about twice as sweet as table sugar) that occurs naturally in honey, as well as fruit, from which it takes its name. It also is found in certain other plants. As a sweetener, it is often more popular than saccharin because its consistency is more like that of ordinary table sugar. However, the caloric difference between fructose and table sugar is insignificant, regardless of how it is prepared. It is also a good deal more expensive than sugar.

Fructose may be safely used (provided the calories are counted) by diabetic patients with good control. It causes a less immediate rise in blood sugar than does sucrose, although it ultimately causes an elevation in blood sugar because the liver converts it to glucose and stores it as glycogen. In some persons fructose may cause flatulence and diarrhea, and its long-term effects are still unclear. Until more is known about fructose, it seems reasonable to use it in moderate amounts, provided you count the calories and do not make it an exclusive substitute for sugar.

Manitol and Sorbitol These naturally occurring sugar alcohols are frequently used as a basic sweetener by manufacturers of candy. Gram for gram, they provide the same number of calories as other caloric sweeteners, but these sugars are absorbed into the blood stream more slowly than glucose so they may cause a less rapid rise in the blood sugar when eaten. Both these substances are half as sweet as sucrose and, when taken in large amounts, can cause diarrhea.

Honey and Syrups Honey has been suggested as a better sweetener since it occurs naturally and contains additional nutriments. It consists of a large amount of glucose and can cause a rapid, excessive elevation in blood sugar when used in excess. Corn syrups are produced by breaking down corn starch into a mixture of maltose, glucose, and other sugar molecules. The amount of these sugars in corn syrup vary widely, and many syrups contain more glucose than usually can be tolerated by diabetics. Since the American Diabetes Association recommends that diabetics restrict sugar consumption, be aware that sugar comes by many names. For example, dextrose, glucose, sucrose, corn syrup, corn syrup solids, sorghum, sugar cane syrup, brown sugar, honey, maple syrup, and molasses all are sugars and should be avoided.

Saccharine and Aspartame The non-sugar sweeteners include saccharine and aspartame. The former was the only artificial, non-nutritive sweetener used in the United States before cyclamates were banned in 1969. It is 300 to 500 times sweeter than sucrose, contains no calories, and does not elevate the blood sugar. The Food and Drug Agency imposed a partial ban of saccharine in 1977 because it had been shown that saccharine caused cancer in laboratory animals. The public objected so strongly that Congress imposed a moritorium on the ban, and now all products containing saccharine are required to display a warning label. Saccharine is frequently used in sugar-free sodas, low-calorie jellies and jams, toppings, and syrups. It can be purchased as a table top sugar substitute and is commercially available in products called Featherweight, saccharine tablets, Sprinkle Sweet, Sweet 'N Low, and so forth.

Aspartame is 200 times sweeter than table sugar, so only very small amounts are required. It is a low caloric sweetener made from two amino acids — aspartic acid and phenylalamine. Since it breaks down at high temperatures, it has been approved for use in drink mixes, cold cereal, gelatins, puddings, dairy products, sugarless gum, and as a table sweetener (Equal). It has no after-taste or known serious side effects, and since it is metabolized as a protein, it does not affect the blood sugar level.

Cooking for Diabetics has been compiled to offer delectable meals that will tantalize the palates of those who undertake the preparation of the wide variety of recipes and menus. They are planned and prepared to provide the proper nourishment with a minimum of harmful "sweets," saturated fats, and cholesterol. The American Diabetes Association diet plan is followed allowing the proper proportions of protein, fats, and carbohydrates. Of course, the culinary delights may be enjoyed by all — diabetics, friends, and family. Each meal has been tested and judged par-excellence. When you are seated with friends to enjoy several of the fine creations from this book, I wish you bon appetite, or just — enjoy.

Practical Tips
for Living with Diabetes

Read, Listen, and Learn All You Can

The news that you or someone you love is a diabetic always comes as a surprise. You may discover the condition as a result of a general physical exam or while hospitalized during a crisis. Either way, it is shocking news. Suddenly someone is sitting before you explaining that now you can only eat this food or that, and that you will have to change your entire style of eating and living.

Let's see now, did she tell me I could lead a normal life, or that I couldn't?

Discovering that you have diabetes does not mark the end of life as you have enjoyed it. With this disease, as with all of life, living is what you make it, and you can live quite comfortably with a change in your dietary needs. Yes, you will have to be more conscious of what you eat, and you will have to take special care of injuries and master the art of blood or urine testing. These are not impossible, or even difficult, skills to learn, but you will need to learn them.

Having diabetes is no cause for despair. You still have much to live for, and your life should remain as rich as ever. You will enjoy your food as much as the next person, and perhaps even more. The diabetic diet is one of the most balanced and healthy one can follow; so don't be afraid of what your doctor or nurse practitioner tells you.

Listen carefully and ask questions. It is important for you to understand your diet, for if you are to cope with it, you will need to understand how it works. The exchange list is there to help, not confuse you. If you find it confusing, then you need to ask questions until you understand how the exchange system works.

To whom can you turn when you need assistance? Your physician is your first resource. Don't be afraid to ask him or her for help when you are confused or afraid. Your doctor also can guide you to the right dietitian or nutritionist who will help you understand what is required and will work with you to develop a well-balanced diet.

Give yourself some credit, too. After all, you have been feeding yourself for quite a few years and you know what you like and dislike in food. Be honest and realistic as you talk with professionals and prepare your diet. Likely as not, if you hated broccoli before your diagnosis, you will continue to hate it. So work with the foods you like, and build on your eating preferences.

Also consider the many books and publications available. Reading is the best way to learn. Study diabetic cookbooks. We think *Cooking For Diabetics* is the best on the market, but whatever sources you use, look carefully at their recipes, compare them with non-diabetic cookbooks, and observe how ingredients are substituted for sugar. You may never read or understand the extensive technical medical information about diabetes that has been published, but you can master the basics.

It also is important to talk with others, particularly family members and friends. Let them know that you have diabetes and that it is going to require some changes in your life. Accept their concern and love, and let them help you. One of the ways you can do this, of course, is to provide them with accurate information. While they will be surprised to learn of your condition, they will not reject you. Most people know at least one person who has diabetes, and you will be surprised at how often someone will tell you about an acquaintance who has diabetes and lives life to the fullest.

Finally, keep an open mind. Don't isolate yourself from what's happening around you. You can lead a productive, active life as a diabetic. The only person who can prevent you from enjoying life is yourself. So don't be your own jailor!

Dealing with Stress

Stress has become a major problem in American society. While some people think stress is good in the sense that it serves to motivate us to action, most researchers and health care professionals would strongly disagree. Stress elevates blood sugar levels and thus can upset the balance you have created in your regimen of diet, exercise, and medication. To restore that balance, you must learn to alleviate the stress in your life.

The first step is to learn how to live with stress. Since it is almost impossible to avoid stress altogether, you must learn to know when you have reached the point that it is affecting you negatively. When this happens, the best thing you can do is simply to take a walk. That's right: walk away. Excuse yourself, get out of the room, get out of the building, take a walk, and breathe deeply while you do it. Once you are relaxed, you will be able to think through what needs to be done to solve the problem and take care of the matter efficiently.

The most effective way to control stress is to plan your activities. Many people are "stressed out" because they have committed to too many things and are always in a rush. To take control of your life, you must eliminate the rush and limit your commitments to a reasonable level.

Plan your life. Before you retire at night, make a list of everything you must do the next day, then set up your priorities and stick to them. If something unexpected arises, include it in your priorities; but do not let it take over your day. Once you have gotten into the habit of planning your time, you will have eliminated your greatest single source of stress.

Another tool for dealing with stress is to give yourself a "time out" period. If you notice that you tend to be under stress at a particular time during the day, incorporate a break before it occurs. If you are unable to schedule a break prior to the time you are vulnerable to stress, do the best you can. What should you do during "time out"? Relax. Lean back in your chair with your feet propped up, read the newspaper, read a book, listen to some music, or take a short walk. Whatever relaxes you, do it!

Other sources of stress reduction include hobbies and exercise. Physical fitness provides you with a sense of well being, increased energy, and greater powers of attention.

Many people find that meaningful religious or spiritual activities aid in alleviating stress. A positive religious experience frequently provides a sense of well-being and serves as a guide through stressful moments.

Whatever actions you take to deal with stress, it is important to remember that a positive attitude is the most helpful resource you can possess. By combining a positive attitude with physical fitness, careful planning, a healthy sense of humor, and meaningful life commitments, you should be able to gain control over stress and enjoy your life.

Eating Out Fast Food Style

People frequently ask us why fast food restaurants have nothing available for the diabetic. Au contraire. In reality, they do offer you something. In general, as a diabetic you can eat at any of the fast food chains, but you will have to choose your foods wisely. While you can't eat the milkshake or cherry pie, you can eat a hamburger or a fish or chicken sandwich. And while French fries are high in fat, many fast food restaurants now offer baked potatoes. It is reported that some fast food establishments are considering offering foods that are low in fat, sugar, salt, and cholesterol. If this ever happens, everyone who controls the amount of these ingredients he or she eats will be grateful for the change.

When eating in fast food restaurants, however, you must always be careful. Just because something comes with the meal is by no means a reason why you should eat it. You can skip the coleslaw that is rich in dressing and sugar, and you can remove the batter from the fish or chicken sandwich and lower the bread content of these foods.

Thankfully, fast food restaurants offer a wide variety of drinks. You can choose from sugar-free soft drinks, ice tea with artificial sweetener, juice, and skim milk.

The most important thing to remember when eating at a fast food restaurant is to be aware of what you can and cannot eat and stay within those guidelines. Better than anyone else, you know when you have eaten the wrong foods or have over-eaten. Think. Be true to your diet, and you can order a fast food meal with confidence.

An Evening Out at the Restaurant

Almost everyone enjoys eating out, especially for those special occasions. What kinds of problems should you expect to confront when enjoying a night on the town?

In general, the following should be true: No more worry should go into dining out than goes into your usual dinner plans. If you know your diet and your allowable portions are clear in mind, you will have very little trouble.

Many diabetics feel more comfortable if they call the restaurant before leaving home. This is a great idea, for it allows you to know what the restaurant has available and allows you time to ask questions beforehand; it also helps you avoid potentially embarrassing situations at a restaurant that is not sensitive to diabetic customers' needs. When you call, you can ask about how they prepare their foods, including whether or not salt and sugar are used.

Perhaps the most immediate problem associated with eating out is the time of the meal. Likely as not, you have a set schedule for eating your evening meal, and this regular mealtime is important. If you know you will be eating earlier or later than usual, keep it in mind as you plan your evening. Usually there are no problems if the meal is served a little early. However, if the meal is served very early (several hours or more), eat lightly and save a bread serving to be eaten at your regular mealtime.

To keep your mealtime at its regular hour, arrive at the restaurant ½ hour early. If it takes even longer for your order to be served, eat a cracker or breadstick. If you know beforehand that your evening meal will be extremely late, eat your bedtime snack at your regular mealtime, and then eat your full meal later.

Choosing food at restaurants is not difficult. Most are happy to prepare foods to your specifications. Broiling meat without the fats or butter should not be a problem, and if the restaurant only offers fried foods, remove the breading. Most restaurants already boil or steam vegetables, so you should ask that sauces, dressings, and butters be served as side orders or in a separate dish so you can determine your own portions.

Traveling Safely

Being a diabetic is no reason for you to feel captive in your home. You can travel safely, and you can make use of all modes of transportation.

Generally, you must give all the usual diabetic considerations when traveling. It is a good idea to keep a check list handy for whenever you prepare to travel. I would suggest the following:

- Insulin
- Syringes
- Swabs
- Blood testing equipment
- Urine testing equipment
- Identification bracelet, cards, and so forth, stating that you are a diabetic and providing your insulin dosage and the name and telephone number of your personal physician
- Extra food for emergency supply
- A letter and extra prescription in case you lose your insulin and/or syringes
- Medicine for vomiting and diarrhea
- Pre-measured glucose tablets

If you are traveling by car, be sure to take into consideration how long it will take you to get there. Likely as not, you hate to stop once you get started. Stopping seems to drag out the drive, so you may attempt to drive longer than you should. This is an extremely dangerous — though attractive — temptation.

If you are driving, you should have about ten grams of carbohydrates every hour to guard against low blood sugar and a possible insulin reaction that could affect your ability to continue driving. Keep handy small portions of fruit, crackers, or raisins. And don't forget the importance of keeping a close watch on your blood glucose levels.

Although it seems so obvious I ought not have to mention it, you must eat your meals and take your insulin or medication at their prescribed times. It is important that you continue to keep your blood levels in balance while you travel.

Traveling by bus or train can create its own problems. Schedules and rest stops are unlikely to match your own schedule. Those inevitable delays create another problem, so be prepared. Take a carry-on snack with you at all times. Keep available at your seat crackers and cheese, a sandwich, or a piece of fruit so you can provide yourself with the needed sugar at your regular mealtimes. One further word of caution: Do not separate yourself from your insulin and syringes. Keep them in your carry-on luggage. Don't be caught without them.

Traveling by plane usually is no problem at all. Thankfully, air travel usually is swift, so long as there are no delays. Even so, you don't want to be caught circling a major airport for hours while your insulin and snacks are in your luggage. Keep these essentials in your carry-on luggage, even when you're flying.

It is important to remember that when using insulin in the air, you are doing so at a lower air pressure than when you are on land. It is wise to insert only half the usual amount of air into your vial when preparing your injection.

I might add that there is another reason for having your insulin on your person and not in your baggage when you travel by air. Trunks and cargo holds are not kept at room temperature at all times. You do not want to render your insulin ineffective by leaving it in hot areas for long periods of time, and often baggage is kept in a very warm environment before it is loaded (or unloaded in some instances). Keep it with you, and there will be no cause for worry.

Changing time zones creates another problem. When you change time zones rapidly as you do when traveling great distances by plane, you need to adjust your dosage. Leave your watch set on "home" time so you can figure how long it has been since your last injection. This can be a very tricky matter, and you need to consult your doctor about how to adjust to new time zones. Discuss this before you leave and make sure you have a definite plan to follow.

If you are traveling overseas, get your shots early. This allows ample time for your system to get over the upsets that usually accompany these injections. If you follow this advice, your own physician who is familiar with your case will be available to help you if a problem develops. Generally, it is wise to plan shots for three to four weeks prior to your scheduled departure.

If you must go through customs and inspection, you should be prepared. Ask your doctor for a letter that explains your diabetes and your need for insulin, medication, syringes, or whatever. Keep the letter on your person, and it will speed you along the customs trail.

If you are traveling in a country with a language other than English, get identification in that language which states that you are a diabetic and gives the details of your medication and dosages. Keep this information with you at all times; generally, it is wise to keep it wherever you keep the rest of your identification (such as in your wallet or billfold). If a medical crisis occurs, this will enable emergency personnel to understand the problem. Some diabetics wear bracelets or necklaces carrying international symbols of identification; wearing them can prevent unnecessary delay in treatment during an emergency.

Finally, although we frequently joke about the subject, you should not drink the water when you travel internationally. The bacteria content in foreign water is different than in your home, and it can cause severe diarrhea and upset of your system. Foods such as milk, cheese, creams, raw leafy vegetables, and fruits should be avoided for the same reasons. Bottled drinks usually are fairly safe, and bottled water should be fine. Drinks served with boiled water, such as coffee, tea, or bouillon, are also safe.

Children and Diabetes

Dealing with a child's medical problems is particularly stressful. You worry, you listen, you act to correct the condition, and you pray it is resolved. This works for most of the medical problems our children face, but diabetes is not cured and it does not go away. Through the right kind of guidance, however, you can watch your child grow up, play in the band, participate in sports, run for homecoming queen, or do whatever he or she chooses. There is no reason for your child to hold back from involvement in any normal activity.

The primary problem diabetic children feel is that of being "different." Children frequently feel as if everyone is staring at them anyway, and diabetic children feel more pressure in this regard than others. They often feel as if people are watching to see if they will turn green or purple when the sugar level "acts up," and it is important for you to educate your child.

First, encourage your child to be open with classmates. It might even be useful to make arrangements for the teacher to schedule a time when diabetes is discussed and the entire class learns what the disease is and what it does. Children are fully capable of understanding this information.

It is also important to let your child know that there will be bad days. You need to remember it, too. These days need to be kept in perspective, however, and one way to help your child is to find a youth support group in your area for children with diabetes and their parents. If after looking you don't find a group, start one. Talk with your pediatrician and get the names of other families that are dealing with diabetes. I will never forget the first meeting I ever attended; it looked like a party. The children seemed relieved to discover they were not so different after all.

You also need to know that there are camps specifically for children with diabetes. These camps usually can be found through the American Diabetes Association. Call or write for their list of summer camps for diabetic children in or near your state.

Parents have a difficult role to play with their diabetic children. Not only do they have to worry about controlling their child's diet, they also must worry constantly about the wide fluctuations in blood sugar that occur from time to time. It is important to remember that in spite of your best efforts to prevent it, these reactions will occur.

Diabetic children are like other children. They love to run, jump, play sports, tease, laugh, and just plain be kids. You need to remember that your child is no different from the next when it comes to activities; he or she is only different when it comes to preparing for the day. Your child takes one more step than the rest in getting started but will run twice as fast to make up for the small delay.

It is important that your child share the responsibility for controlling his diabetes. Granted, it seems like a heavy load to give to a child, and you will want to take his or her age and level of responsibility into consideration. You should not force your child to take responsibility; you should offer the opportunity to become involved.

For instance, you can let your child help pick out foods based on likes and dislikes. Let him figure out whether they are high or low in sugar. You also can let your child pick where his next injection site should be, wipe the area with alcohol before the injection, and give his own shots, depending on his capabilities. Some children will want to be involved in blood testing, including interpreting the results.

In short, children are able to cope and deal with life situations as well as adults, and sometimes even better. They tend to see life as it is, so you should do them a favor and give them the honest, straight truth. They can handle it.

We have found that charts can serve as helpful reminders for children. They aid in seeing what needs to be done, and they provide a handy reference tool for remembering what tasks have been completed. In being able to refer to their chart regularly, children can feel in control of their diabetes and in control of their lives. I would recommend that you use colorful stickers or stamps for keeping track of what has and has not been done. They are a lot more fun than merely checking off each task with a pen or pencil.

A sample chart is given below:

	Out of bed at 6:45 am	Checked blood or urine	Results	Gave own shot	Dose amount
Sunday					
Monday					
Tuesday					
Wednesday					
Thursday					
Friday					
Saturday					

A Guide to Meal Planning

Reading the Labels

The first place to look for the nutritional information about food is on the label, and the proper time to study the label is while you are at the grocery store. Unfortunately, labels don't always give you the information you need and can be quite confusing. It is important that you learn to recognize the following names for sugar:

Fructose: This is the simple sugar found naturally in fruits. Some diabetics are able to use it, but you should talk with your dietitian about how much you are able to use.

Sorbitol: This is an alcohol sugar that is absorbed very slowly. You need to talk with your dietitian about how much sorbitol you are able to use.

Xylitol: This was used in sugarless mints and gum because it caused fewer dental cavities than sucrose. It was taken off the market when it was found to cause cancer in laboratory animals.

All of the above sugar substitutes have calories. Those following do not have calories.

Saccharine: This non-nutritive sweetener is available in tablet, powder, and liquid forms. When heated, it takes on a metallic taste; so its use is limited to recipes that are not heated.

Aspartame: Also known as Equal, it is found in powder and tablet forms. "Nutra Sweet" is the bulk form of aspartame used in food products such as puddings, gelatin, beverage mixes, and soft drinks. Aspartame loses some of its sweetness when heated.

When looking at a label, you should check the ingredients list first. The list provides helpful information, particularly if you keep in mind that they are listed in order of highest to lowest amount by weight. If you are trying to avoid sugar, observe how far down the listing the sugar appears.

Also be careful of claims made on the label in bold type. This includes such words as *Lite, Reduced, Light, Low calorie,* and so forth. Generally these words have hidden meanings. *Lite* may mean that the color is light, that the product weighs less than usual, or that it has more water than traditionally is the case. *Reduced* may also mean many things: reduced price, reduced additives, reduced weight. All this means very little in gathering information to use in watching your diet.

So read those labels and the nutritional breakdowns carefully; then you will know what is in the food you buy. Compare the ingredients and nutritional information with other products, and then you will be able to see what the words designed to catch your attention really mean.

Meal Planning

The following menu plans rely upon the American Diabetes Association's exchange lists. They are available through the American Diabetes Association in your state or local area, as well as through your physician's office.

Included are menu plans for diets allowing several different levels of caloric intake: 1,000, 1,200, 1,500, 1,800, 2,000, 2,500, and 3,000 calories per day. Though these diets may look confusing at first glance, the more you use the diet the more sense it will make. Soon the planning process will become so familiar that you will only use the exchange list for occasional reference.

1,000 Calorie Daily Food Allowances. (This is not a recommended caloric intake and is only included here because occasionally it is recommended. This diet should only be used under a physician's direct care and guidance.)

Breakfast
½ fruit exchange . . . . List 3
1 bread exchange . . . . List 4
1 medium fat meat exchange . . . . . List 5
1 fat exchange . . . . List 6
1 milk exchange (no fat) . . . . List 1

Lunch
1 lean meat exchange . . . . List 5
1 bread exchange . . . . List 4
1 vegetable exchange . . . . List 2
1 fruit exchange . . . . List 3
1 fat exchange . . . . List 6

Dinner
2 lean meat exchanges . . . . List 5
1 bread exchange . . . . List 4

1 vegetable exchange . . . . List 2
Free vegetable(s) as desired . . . . . List 2°
1 fruit exchange . . . . List 3
1 fat exchange . . . . List 6
1 milk exchange . . . . List 1

Bedtime Snack
½ bread exchange . . . . List 4
½ milk exchange (no fat) . . . . List 1

Provides
Carbohydrates . . . . 124 grams
Protein . . . . 59 grams
Fat . . . . 29 grams

1,200 Calorie Daily Food Allowances

Breakfast
1 fruit exchange	List 3
1 bread exchange	List 4
1 medium fat meat exchange	List 5
1 fat exchange	List 6
1 milk exchange (no fat)	List 1

Lunch
1 lean meat exchange	List 5
2 bread exchanges	List 4
1 vegetable exchange	List 2
2 fruit exchanges	List 3
2 fat exchanges	List 6

Dinner
2 lean meat exchanges	List 5
1 bread exchange	List 4
1 vegetable exchange	List 2
Free vegetable(s) as desired	List 2*
2 fruit exchanges	List 3
1 fat exchange	List 6

Bedtime Snack
1 milk exchange (no fat)	List 1
1 fruit exchange	List 4

Provides
Carbohydrates	169 grams
Protein	57 grams
Fat	34 grams

1,500 Calorie Daily Food Allowances

Breakfast
2 fruit exchanges	List 3
1 bread exchange	List 4
1 medium fat meat exchange	List 5
2 fat exchanges	List 6
1 milk exchange (no fat)	List 1

Lunch
2 lean meat exchanges	List 5
1 vegetable exchange	List 2
2 fat exchanges	List 6
2 bread exchanges	List 4
2 fruit exchanges	List 3

Dinner
2 lean meat exchanges	List 5
2 bread exchanges	List 4
1 vegetable exchange	List 2
Free vegetable(s) as desired	List 2*
2 fruit exchanges	List 3
2 fat exchanges	List 6

Bedtime Snack
1 bread exchange	List 4
1 milk exchange (no fat)	List 1

Provides
Carbohydrates	214 grams
Protein	66 grams
Fat	44 grams

1,800 Calorie Daily Food Allowances

Breakfast

2 fruit exchanges	List 3
2 bread exchanges	List 4
1 medium fat meat exchange	List 5
2 fat exchanges	List 6
1 milk exchange (no fat)	List 1

Lunch

2 lean meat exchanges	List 5
1 vegetable exchange	List 2
2 fat exchanges	List 6
2 bread exchanges	List 4
2 fruit exchanges	List 3
½ milk exchange (no fat)	List 1

Dinner

3 lean meat exchanges	List 5
2 bread exchanges	List 4
2 vegetable exchanges	List 2
Free vegetable(s) as desired	List 2*
2 fruit exchanges	List 3
2 fat exchanges	List 6

Bedtime Snack

1 bread exchange	List 4
1 lean meat exchange	List 5
1 milk exchange (no fat)	List 1
1 fruit exchange	List 4
1 fat exchange	List 6

Provides

Carbohydrates	254 grams
Protein	73 grams
Fat	54 grams

2,000 Calorie Daily Food Allowances

Breakfast

2 fruit exchanges	List 3
2 bread exchanges	List 4
1 medium fat meat exchange	List 5
2 fat exchanges	List 6
1 milk exchange (no fat)	List 1

Lunch

3 lean meat exchanges	List 5
1 vegetable exchange	List 2
2 fat exchanges	List 6
2 bread exchanges	List 4
Vegetable(s) as desired	List 2*
2 fruit exchanges	List 3
1 milk exchange (no fat)	List 1

Dinner

3 lean meat exchanges	List 5
3 bread exchanges	List 4
2 vegetable exchanges	List 2
Free vegetable(s) as desired	List 2*
2 fruit exchanges	List 3
2 fat exchanges	List 6

Bedtime Snack

1 bread exchange	List 4
1 fruit exchange	List 3
1 milk exchange (no fat)	List 5
1 fat exchange	List 6

Provides

Carbohydrates	284 grams
Protein	86 grams
Fat	57 grams

2,500 Calorie Daily Food Allowances

Breakfast
2 fruit exchanges	List 3
4 bread exchanges	List 4
1 medium fat meat exchange	List 5
3 fat exchanges	List 6
1 milk exchange (no fat)	List 1

3 vegetable exchanges	List 2
Free vegetable(s) as desired	List 2*
2 fruit exchanges	List 3
3 fat exchanges	List 6

Lunch
2 lean meat exchanges	List 5
4 bread exchanges	List 4
4 fat exchanges	List 6
2 vegetable exchanges	List 2
2 fruit exchanges	List 3

Bedtime Snack
1 bread exchange	List 4
1 fat exchange	List 6
1 milk exchange (no fat)	List 6
2 fruit exchanges	List 4

Dinner
2 lean meat exchanges	List 5
4 bread exchanges	List 4

Provides
Carbohydrates	364 grams
Protein	100 grams
Fat	72 grams

3,000 Calorie Daily Food Allowances

Breakfast
2 fruit exchanges	List 3
4 bread exchanges	List 4
1 medium fat meat exchange	List 5
4 fat exchanges	List 6
1 milk exchange (no fat)	List 1

Lunch
2 lean meat exchanges	List 5
4 bread exchanges	List 4
4 fat exchanges	List 6
3 vegetable exchanges	List 2
2 fruit exchanges	List 3

Mid-morning Snack
1 fruit exchange	List 4
1 fat exchange	List 6

Mid-afternoon Snack
1 fat exchange	List 6
1 bread exchange	List 4
1 fruit exchange	List 3

Dinner

2 lean meat exchanges	List 5
4 bread exchanges	List 4
3 vegetable exchanges	List 2
Free vegetable(s) as desired	List 2*
2 fruit exchanges	List 3
4 fat exchanges	List 6
1 milk exchange (no fat)	List 1

Bedtime Snack

2 lean meat exchanges	List 5
2 bread exchanges	List 4
2 fat exchanges	List 6
1 milk exchange (no fat)	List 1
1 fruit exchange	List 4

Provides

Carbohydrates	429 grams
Protein	111 grams
Fat	92 grams

Working with the Exchange System

Diabetic diets are usually set by the use of the exchange list developed in 1950 by the American Diabetes Association, the American Dietetic Association, and the Chronic Disease Program of the United States Public Health Service. This listing of foods enables diabetics to choose within the listings food for their daily needs. The exchange list takes into consideration the chemical components of foods, such as carbohydrates, proteins, fats, and calories. This list is important for all diabetics, for it helps them to maintain blood sugar levels by adequately picking nutritious foods for their meals without overeating.

Your personal physician or dietitian is the person who should control how you use the exchange list. This means that he or she has told you either how many calories you are permitted to eat or how many carbohydrates you are allowed within a twenty-four-hour period. Your diet counselor has set standards, such as two bread exchanges for your morning meal. You can translate this instruction by looking at the exchange list for breads and choosing what those breads will include. This could mean, for instance, that you might eat ½ cup of bran flakes and a slice of whole wheat bread; they are equivalent to two bread exchanges.

Lately we have noticed a trend toward counting carbohydrates, rather than counting calories. In following this method, the diet counselor or physician allows a certain number of carbohydrates in the daily meal (including the number allowed per meal and for snacks) and then provides lists of foods and their carbohydrate levels. This, too, is a useful way to plan your daily diet. Your physician will advise you regarding which plan is right for you.

Because of the two dietary tools available for planning the diabetic diet (and of other restricted diet plans), we have included within this book both the approved exchange list and a chemical breakdown of foods that includes the carbohydrates, proteins, fats, cholesterol, sodium, calories, and percentage of calories from fat in each recipe. This has been done to better inform you of the nutritional value of each recipe and to help you use the recipes according to the guidelines set for you.

Diabetic Exchange Lists

General Rules and Guidelines
- Food should be weighed and measured. Standard measuring cups and spoons will be required. Measure cooked foods after they are cooked.
- Meats should be baked, broiled, roasted, or boiled. Do not fry foods unless fat is allowed in the meal.
- Avoid sugar, candy, honey, jam, jelly, most cakes, pies and cookies, syrups, pastries, and regular soft drinks.
- Eat meals about the same time every day. Eat the amounts on the meal plan and do not skip meals.

List 1 ▪ Milk Exchanges

One exchange of milk contains 12 grams of carbohydrate, 8 grams of protein, a trace of fat, and 90 calories.

Non-fat fortified milk

Skim or non-fat milk (½% or 1%)	1 cup
Powdered (non-fat dry before adding liquid)	⅓ cup
Canned, evaporated made from skim milk	½ cup
Buttermilk, from skim milk	1 cup
Alba 66 or 77	1 envelope
Yogurt made from skim milk, plain (Frozen or flavored yogurts contain sugar and are not recommended)	1 cup

Low-fat fortified milk

2% fat fortified milk (Omit 1 fat exchange)	1 cup

Yogurt made from 2% milk, plain (Omit 1 fat exchange)	1 cup

Whole milk
(Omit 2 fat exchanges)

Canned, evaporated made from whole milk	½ cup
Buttermilk made from whole milk	1 cup
Yogurt made from whole milk (plain)	1 cup
Eggnog, non-alcoholic (Omit 1½ bread exchanges)	1 cup
Custard	½ cup

List 2 ▪ Vegetable Exchanges

One vegetable exchange contains about 5 grams of carbohydrate, 2 grams of protein, and 25 calories.

This list shows the kinds of vegetables to use for one vegetable exchange. One exchange equals ½ cup cooked or 1 cup raw.

Artichoke (Globe or Jerusalem)
Asparagus
Bamboo shoots
Bean sprouts
Beets
Broccoli
Brussels sprouts
Cabbage*
Carrots
Cauliflower
Celery*
Chinese cabbage*
Eggplant
Green pepper
Greens:
  Beet
  Chards
  Collards
  Dandelion
  Kale
  Mustard
  Spinach*
  Turnip
Kohlrabi
Mixed vegetables (⅓ cup)
Mushrooms*

Okra
Onions
Pea pods (Snow peas)
Rhubarb
Rutabaga
Sauerkraut
String beans, green or wax
Squash:
  Cocozelle
  Crookneck
  Straightneck
  Summer
  Zucchini*
Tomatoes
Tomato catsup (1 tablespoon)
Tomato juice
Tomato paste (2 tablespoons)
Tomato puree (¼ cup)
Tomato sauce (not barbecue)
Turnips
Vegetable juice cocktail
Water chestnuts (4)
Green onion*
*One cup of these vegetables raw is considered a free food.

The following raw vegetables may be used as desired:

Chicory
Cucumbers
Endive
Escarole
Lettuce
Hot peppers

Parsley
Pimiento
Radishes
Romaine
Watercress
Pickles, dill

List 3 • Fruit Exchanges

One fruit exchange contains 15 grams of carbohydrate and 60 calories.

Canned fruits may be packed in water or in their own juices. If packed in juice, the fruit should be eaten without the juice, or the calories in the juice must be counted as another fruit serving.

This list shows the kinds and amounts of fruits to use for one fruit exchange.*

Apple	1 small	Melon:	
Apple juice	½ cup	Cataloupe	
Applesauce,		(5 inches across)	⅓ small or 1 cup
unsweetened	½ cup	Honeydew	⅛ medium or
Apricots, canned	4 medium halves		1 cup
Apricots, fresh	4 medium	Watermelon	1¼ cups
Apricots, dried	7 halves	Nectarine	1 cup
Banana		Orange	1 small
(9 inches long)	½ small	Orange juice	½ cup
Berries:		Orange sections	½ cup
Blackberries	¾ cup	Papaya	1 cup
Blueberries	¾ cup	Peach	1 medium
Raspberries	1 cup	Peach, canned	½ cup or
Strawberries	1¼ cup		2 medium halves
Cherries	12 large	Pear	1 small
Cherries,		Pear, canned	½ cup or
red sour pitted	½ cup		2 medium halves
Cider	½ cup	Persimmon, native	2 medium
Dates	2½ medium	Pineapple, canned	⅓ cup
Figs, fresh	2	Pineapple juice	½ cup
Figs, dried	1½	Pineapple, raw	¾ cup
Fruit cocktail	½ cup	Plums	2 medium
Grapefruit	½	Prune juice	⅓ cup
Grapefruit juice	½ cup	Prunes	3 medium
Grapefruit sections	¾ cup	Raisins	2 tablespoons
Grape juice	⅓ cup	Rhubarb, fresh or	
Grapes	15	unsweetened	
Guava	½ medium	frozen*	1 cup
Kiwi (large)	1	Tangerine (2½ inches	
Mango	½ small	across)	2

*Cranberries: ½ cup may be used as desired if no sugar is added
*Rhubarb, unsweetened (½ cup), is a free food.

Other Juices: Unsweetened fruit juices are preferred as fruit exchanges. Avoid fruit drinks and artificial fruit juices.

Cranberry juice cocktail	⅓ cup	Lime juice	½ cup
Cranapple juice (low calorie)	1 cup	Orange-grapefruit juice	½ cup
Cranberry juice (low calorie)	¾ cup	Tomato juice	1 cup
Lemon juice	½ cup	Vegetable juice cocktail	1 cup

List 4 ▪ Starch Exchanges

One starch exchange contains 15 grams of carbohydrates, 3 grams of protein, a trace of fat, and 80 calories.

Bread

White (including French and Italian)	1 slice	Pancake (Omit 1 fat exchange)	1
Whole wheat	1 slice	Waffle (Omit 1 fat exchange)	1
Diet bread (35 calories per slice)	2 slices	Plain roll	1
Rye or pumpernickel	1 slice	Frankfurter roll	½
Raisin	1 slice	Hamburger roll	½
Bagel, small	½	Dried bread crumbs	3 tablespoons
Biscuit, 2-inch diameter (Omit 1 fat exchange)	1	Bread dressing (Omit 1 fat exchange)	¼ cup)
Cornbread (1x2x2 inches)	1	Bread sticks, 9-inch	2
Croissants (Omit 1½ starch exchange and 2 fat exchanges)	1	Taco shell, 6-inch (Omit 1 fat exchange)	1
French toast (Omit 1 starch exchange and ½ meat exchange)	1 slice	Tortilla, 6-inch	1
Muffin, small English	½	*Cereals and Starches*	
Muffin, plain, blueberry, or bran (Omit 1 fat exchange)	1	Bran flakes	½ cup
		Granola types (Omit 1 fat exchange)	¼ cup
		Other ready-to-eat cereals, unsweetened	¾ cup

Puffed cereals, unsweetened	1½ cup	Saltines	6
Cereal, cooked	½ cup	Soda, 2½ inches square	4
Grits, cooked	½ cup	Triscuits (Omit 1 fat exchange)	5
Hominy, cooked	½ cup	Vanilla wafer (Omit 1 fat exchange)	6
Tapioca, granulated	2 tablespoons		
Rice or barley, cooked	⅓ cup		
Rice, long grain wild	½ cup	Wheat Thins (Omit 1 fat exchange)	12
Chinese noodles (Omit 1 fat exchange)	½ cup		

Starchy Vegetables

Pasta:	
Spaghetti, cooked	½ cup
Noodles, cooked	½ cup
Macaroni, cooked	½ cup

Dried beans and peas, cooked	⅓ cup
Lima beans	½ cup
Beans, baked canned	¼ cup
Popcorn, popped (no fat added)	3 cups
Corn	⅓ cup
Corn on the cob	½ ear
Cornmeal, dry	2½ tablespoons
Corn, cream style	¼ cup
Cornstarch	2 tablespoons
Parsnips	⅔ cup
Flour	2½ tablespoons
Matzo meal	3 tablespoons
Peas, green (canned or frozen)	½ cup
Wheat germ	3 tablespoons
Potato, white	1 small
Crackers:	
Animal crackers	8
Potato, mashed	½ cup
Arrowroot	3
Potato, au gratin (Omit 1 fat exchange)	½ cup
Cheese tidbits (Omit 1 fat exchange)	3
Potato, cottage fries (Omit 1 fat exchange)	2 ounces
Croutons, plain	2 tablespoons
Potato, hash browns (Omit 1 fat exchange)	½ cup
Graham, 2½ inches square	3
Matzoth, 4x6 inches	¾ ounces
Potato, scalloped (Omit 1 fat exchange)	½ cup
Melba toast	10 rounds
Oyster	24
Tater-tots (Omit 1 fat exchange)	½ cup
Pretzels (3⅛ inches long x ⅛ inch diameter)	25
Pumpkin	¾ cup
Ritz, HiHo (Omit 1 fat exchange)	6
Winter squash, acorn or butternut	¾ cup
Rusk	2
Yam or sweet potato	⅓ cup
Rye wafer	4

List 5 ▪ Meat Exchanges

Lean Meat Exchanges

Each portion supplies approximately 7 grams of protein, 3 grams of fat, and 55 calories. Trim all visible fat.

Beef

Baby beef, very lean	1 ounce
Chipped beef	1 ounce
Chuck	1 ounce
Filet mignon	1 ounce
Flank steak	1 ounce
Plate ribs	1 ounce
Plate skirt steak	1 ounce
Round, bottom or top	1 ounce
Round, lean ground (90%)	1 ounce
Rump, all cuts	1 ounce
Stew meat	1 ounce
Tenderloin	1 ounce

Pork

Leg, whole rump, center shank	1 ounce
Ham, smoked (center slices)	1 ounce

Veal

Leg	1 ounce
Loin	1 ounce
Rib	1 ounce
Shank	1 ounce
Shoulder	1 ounce

Poultry

Capon (without skin)	1 ounce
Chicken (without skin)	1 ounce
Cornish hen (without skin)	1 ounce
Guinea hen (without skin)	1 ounce
Pheasant (without skin)	1 ounce
Turkey (without skin)	1 ounce

Fish

Any fresh or frozen fish	1 ounce
Clams	2 ounces
Crab	2 ounces
Herring, uncreamed or smoked	1 ounce
Lobster	2 ounces
Oysters	6 medium
Salmon, canned	¼ cup
Sardines, drained	2
Scallops	2 ounces
Shrimp	2 ounces
Tuna, water packed	¼ cup

Game

Duck (without skin)	1 ounce
Goose (without skin)	1 ounce
Pheasant (without skin)	1 ounce
Rabbit	1 ounce
Squirrel	1 ounce
Venison (without skin)	1 ounce

Lowfat cheeses

Cottage cheese (1% or 2%)	¼ cup
Farmer's cheese	1 ounce
Light N Lively	1 ounce
Lite-Line	1 ounce
Parmesan, grated	2 tablespoons
Slimline, Weight Watchers Lo Fat Cheese	1 ounce
St. Otho	1 ounce
Cheese containing less than 5% butterfat	1 ounce

Dried beans and peas

Chick peas (2 starches and 1 meat exchange)	1 cup	Navy beans (2 starches and 1 meat exchange)	1 cup
Cowpeas (2 starches and 1 meat exchange)	1 cup	Pinto beans (2 starches and 1 meat exchange)	1 cup
Garbanzo beans (2 starches and 1 meat exchange)	1 cup	Soy beans (2 starches and 1 meat exchange)	1 cup
Kidney beans (2 starches and 1 meat exchange)	1 cup	Split peas (2 starches and 1 meat exchange)	1 cup
Lentils (2 starches and 1 meat exchange)	1 cup	Egg Substitutes, low cholesterol	¼ cup
Lima beans (2 starches and 1 meat exchange)	1 cup	95% fat free luncheon meats	1 ounce

Medium-fat meat exchanges

Each portion supplies approximately 7 grams of protein, 5 grams of fat, and 75 calories. Trim off all visible fat.

Beef		*Pork*	
Chuck roast	1 ounce	Boiled ham	1 ounce
Corned beef (canned)	1 ounce	Boston butt	1 ounce
Ground beef (15% fat)	1 ounce	Canadian bacon	1 ounce
Ground round	1 ounce	Loin (all cuts tenderloin)	1 ounce
New York strip steak	1 ounce	Pork chops	1 ounce
Porterhouse steak	1 ounce	Shoulder arm (picnic)	1 ounce
Pot roast	1 ounce	Shoulder blade	1 ounce
Rib eye steak	1 ounce		
Rib roast	1 ounce	*Lamb*	
Sirloin tip roast	1 ounce	Chops	1 ounce
T-bone steak	1 ounce	Leg	1 ounce
Tongue (3x2x⅛ inches)	1 slice	Roast	1 ounce
Veal		Liver, heart, kidney, and sweetbreads (These are high in cholesterol.)	1 ounce
Ground or cubed	1 ounce		
Veal cutlet	1 ounce		

Cheese

Casino	1 ounce
Cheez Whiz	1 ounce
Cheezola	1 ounce
Cottage cheese, creamed	¼ cup
Hickory Farms Longhorn Lyte	1 ounce
Hickory Farms Smokie Lyte	1 ounce
Mozzarella	1 ounce
Neufchatel	1 ounce
Ricotta	1 ounce
Skim American cheese	1 ounce
Velveeta	1 ounce

Tofu	4 ounces
Egg (High in cholesterol)	1

Poultry

Duck, wild	1 ounce

Fish

Anchovies	9 thin fillets
Anchovy paste	2 tablespoons
Caviar	1 tablespoon
Fish sticks (Omit 1 fat exchange)	4 sticks
Mackerel	1 ounce
Smelt	1 ounce
Trout	1 ounce

High-fat Meat Exchanges

Each portion contains approximately 7 grams of protein, 8 grams of fat, and 100 calories. Trim off all visible fat.

Beef

Brisket	1 ounce
Club steak	1 ounce
Corned beef	1 ounce
Ground beef (more than 20% fat)	1 ounce
Hamburger (commercial)	1 ounce
Chuck (ground commercial)	1 ounce
Rib roasts	1 ounce
Rib steaks	1 ounce

Lamb

Breast	1 ounce

Pork

Country style ham	1 ounce
Loin (back ribs)	1 ounce
Pig's feet	4 ounces
Pork (ground)	1 ounce
Sausage	1 ounce
Sizzlean	3
Spare ribs	1 ounce
Vienna sausages	3 small

Luncheon meats

Bologna	1 ounce
Braunschweiger	1 ounce
Deviled ham	1 ounce

Frankfurters, chicken or turkey	1	Spam	1 ounce
		Treet	1 ounce
Frankfurters, beef or pork (Omit 1 fat exchange)	1	*Cheese*	
Liverwurst	1 ounce	All regular cheese, such as	
Pastrami	1 ounce	American, bleu, Cheddar,	
Pepperoni	1 ounce	Monterey, Swiss	1 ounce
Polish sausage	1 ounce		
Salami	1 ounce	Peanut butter	1 tablespoon

List 6 ▪ Fat Exchanges

One fat exchange contains 5 grams of fat and 45 calories. Fats listed below are recommended for low fat diets.

Avocado (4 inches in diameter)***	⅛	Oil:	
		Corn	1 teaspoon
Margarine, soft, tub, or stick	1 teaspoon	Cottonseed	1 teaspoon
		Olive***	1 teaspoon
Margarine**	2 teaspoons	Peanut***	1 teaspoon
Margarine, diet	1 tablespoon	Safflower	1 teaspoon
Nuts:		Soy	1 teaspoon
Almonds***	6 whole	Sunflower	1 teaspoon
Peanuts***	20 small	Olives***	5 small
Pecans***	2 large whole		
Walnuts	2 whole		
Other	1 tablespoon		

Fats listed below are not recommended for low fat diets.

Bacon, crisp	1 slice	Coconut, fresh or un-sweetened, shredded	2 tablespoons
Bacon fat	1 teaspoon		
Butter	1 teaspoon	Coffee whitener (liquid)	2 tablespoons
Chitterlings	2 tablespoons		

Coffee whitener (powder)	4 teaspoons	Pepitas (hulled pumpkin seeds)	1 tablespoon
Cracklins	1 rounded teaspoon	Salad dressing, mayonnaise type****	2 teaspoons
Cream cheese	1 tablespoon		
Cream, heavy	1 tablespoon		
Cream, light	2 tablespoons	Salad dressing, reduced calorie mayonnaise type	1 tablespoon
Cream, sour	2 tablespoons		
Gravy	2 tablespoons		
French dressing***	1 tablespoon	Salad dressing, reduced calorie*	2 tablespoons
Italian dressing***	1 tablespoon		
Lard	1 teaspoon	Salt pork	¾-inch cube
Margarine, regular stick	1 teaspoon	Sesame seeds	1 tablespoon
		Sunflower seeds, hulled	1 tablespoon
Mayonnaise****	1 teaspoon		
Mayonnaise, reduced calorie	1 tablespoon		

   * Free food.

  ** Made with corn, cottonseed, safflower, soy, sunflower only.

 *** Fat content is primarily monounsaturated.

**** If made with corn, cottonseed, safflower, soy, or sunflower oil, may be used on fat modified diet.

Free Foods

Free foods are relatively low in calories, less than 15 to 20 per serving. Limit free foods to a total of 50 to 60 calories per day divided between meals and snacks. Do not eat them all at one time.

Bacon bits	2 teaspoons	Catsup	1 tablespoon
Broth, fat-free	No limit	Chili sauce	1 tablespoon
Butter Buds	1 ounce	Club soda	No limit
Carbonated beverages, sugar-free	No limit	Cocoa, unsweetened dry	1 tablespoon

Coffee or tea, unsweetened	No limit	Lemon or lemon juice	Amount not to exceed 20 calories
Cool Whip	2 tablespoons	Mustard	1 tablespoon
Diet salad dressings	Amount not to exceed 20 calories	Non-nutritive sweeteners	No limit
Diet gelatin	Amount not to exceed 20 calories	Onion	No limit
		Soy sauce	1 tablespoon
Diet maple syrup	Amount not to exceed 20 calories	Taco sauce	1 tablespoon
		Tomato paste	1 tablespoon
Dill pickle	1	Vegetable pan spray	No limit
Dream Whip	2 tablespoons	Vinegar	No limit
Herbs, seasonings, and spices	No limit	Worcestershire sauce	1 tablespoon
Jams, jellies, artificially sweetened	Amount not to exceed 20 calories	Yogurt, plain	2 tablespoons
Kool-Aid, unsweetened	No limit		

Soups

	Amount	Exchanges
Bean with bacon	1 cup	1½ starch, 1 fat
Beef broth	No limit	
Beef noodle	1 cup	½ starch, ½ meat
Chicken and dumplings	1 cup	½ starch, ½ meat, ½ fat
Chicken, Cream of	1 cup	½ starch, ½ meat, ½ fat
Chicken noodle	1 cup	½ starch, ½ fat
Chicken vegetable	1 cup	½ starch, ½ fat
Chicken with rice	1 cup	½ starch, ½ fat
Clam chowder, Manhattan style	1 cup	1 vegetable, ½ starch, ½ fat
French onion	1 cup	½ starch, ½ fat
Minestrone	1 cup	1 vegetable, ½ starch, ½ fat
Potato, cream of (made with skim milk)	1 cup	½ milk, ½ starch, ½ fat
Tomato	1 cup	1 starch, ½ fat
Turkey noodle	1 cup	½ starch, ½ fat
Vegetable	1 cup	1 vegetable, ½ starch, ½ fat

Special Foods and Snacks

These are regular sweetened foods, with the exception of the low calorie pudding. These foods should be used only for special occasions with the advice of a physician or dietitian.

Food	Amount	Exchange
Cake, angel (plain)	1/12 cake	2 starches
Cake, pound	3-inch square	2 starches, 2 fats
Cake, sponge	1½-inch square	1 starch
Cheetos	¾ ounce	1 starch, 1 fat
Chocolate chip cookies	2	1 starch
Chocolate or vanilla pudding	⅓ cup	1 starch, 1 fat
Cinnamon Crisps	4	1 starch
Custard, baked	½ cup	1 starch, 1 fat
Dairy Queen frozen dessert	½ cup	2 starches, 1 fat
Doughnuts, plain	1 small	1 starch, 1 fat
Fritos	1 ounce	1 starch, 2 fats
Gelatin, sweetened	½ cup	1 starch
Granola bar, plain	1	1 starch, 1 fat
Honey	2 teaspoons	1 fruit
Ice cream, plain flavors	½ cup	1 starch, 2 fats
Ice cream, soft serve	½ cup	1 starch, 1 fat
Ice milk	½ cup	1 starch, 1 fat
Jelly beans	6	1 fruit
Lifesavers	5	1 fruit
Marshmallows	2	1 fruit
Nuts:		
Cashews	¼ cup	1 meat, 2 fats
Mixed	¼ cup	1 meat, 2 fats
Onion rings	2 ounces	1 starch, 1 fat
Popsicles	½ ounce	1 fruit
Potato chips	1 ounce	1 starch, 2 fats
Pretzels	¾ ounce	1 starch
Pudding (low calorie) made with skim milk	½ cup	1 starch
Sherbet	½ cup	2 starches
Weight Watchers frozen dessert	½ cup	1 starch, 1 fat

Combination Foods

	Amount	Exchanges
Beef stew	1 cup	2 starches, 2 meats, 1 fat
Beef stroganoff	1 cup	2 starches, 2 meats, 1 fat
Cannelloni	4 stuffed noodles	4 meats, 2 vegetables, 1 fat
Chicken Tetrazzini	1 cup	1½ starches, 2 meats
Chili Con Carne with beans	1 cup	2 meats, 2 starches, 2 fats
Lasagne	1 serving (3x4 inches)	1 starch, 1 vegetable, 2½ meats
Macaroni and cheese	1 cup	2 starches, 1 meat, 1 fat
Manicotti	2 shells	2 vegetables, 3 meats, 2 fats
Ravioli with beef/cheese	1 cup	2 starches, 1 vegetable, 1 meat 1 fat

A Sample 2,000 Calorie Diet Menu for One Day

It is not unusual for those just beginning to cook and plan menus for diabetics to experience frustration or confusion when faced with lists of exchanges and menu plans. It seems so complicated at first. For that reason, we have shown below how to work with the calorie and exchange systems; for sake of illustration, we have chosen a 2,000 calorie per day diet.

In the example given, the number of calories has been the controlling factor. Your doctor or dietician may prefer for you to plan your meals according to carbohydrates or to follow the exchange lists closely. Regardless, by careful planning and attention to detail, you can provide nutritious, interesting meals filled with delicious food.

All of the foods included in this menu appear in Cooking for Diabetics. Enjoy!

Breakfast

6-ounce glass of Fruity Good Morning Drink	106 calories	½ milk, 1 fruit
1 Oat Bran Banana Muffin	173 calories	2 bread, 1 fat
1 8-ounce glass skim milk	60 calories	1 milk
½ broiled grapefruit	60 calories	½ fruit
1 ounce low cholesterol cheese	75 calories	1 medium lean meat

Lunch

Fluffy Orange Yogurt Salad	118 calories	2 fruit
Family Beef Stew	244 calories	½ vegetable, 1 bread, 2 meat, 1 fat
Fall Apple Coffee	109 calories	2 fruit
Scottish Oat Bran Toast	107 calories	1 bread, 1 fat
½ cup skim milk	60 calories	1 milk

Dinner

Refreshing Chilled Strawberry Soup	92 calories	2 fruit
Stuffed Chicken Breasts	266 calories	½ bread, 3½ meat, 2 fat
Spaghetti Squash and Vegetables	57 calories	3½ vegetable
Yogurt Drop Biscuits	63 calories	1 bread
2 Russian Tea Cakes	150 calories	1 bread, 2 fats
Iced tea	0 calories	free

Snack

1 slice applesauce cake	251 calories	2 bread, 2 fats

Total for day: 1,991 calories

Appetizers

Colonial Orange Spiced Walnuts

TWENTY-FOUR TABLESPOONFULS

1 .3-ounce package orange sugar-free gelatin
2 cups boiling water
1½ cups walnut halves
½ tablespoon grated orange rind
¼ teaspoon cinnamon
⅛ teaspoon ginger
⅛ teaspoon cloves
   Pinch of nutmeg

*Exchange Values
Per Tablespoon:*
1 Fat

50 Calories
(83% from Fat)
1.5gm Carbohydrates
1.4gm Protein
4.6gm Fat
0mg Cholesterol
2mg Sodium
45mg Potassium

*I*n a heavy skillet combine the gelatin and boiling water. Add the remaining ingredients and bring to a boil again over medium heat, stir until most of the liquid is evaporated. Drain on a paper towel. Spread on a cookie sheet to cool.

Garlic and Parmesan Pecans

THIRTY-TWO TABLESPOONFULS

2   tablespoons liquid margarine
½   teaspoon garlic powder
½   teaspoon brown mustard
½   teaspoon Worcestershire sauce
2   cups pecan halves and large pieces
⅓   cup grated Parmesan cheese

*H*eat the margarine in a medium skillet until melted. Stir in the garlic powder, mustard, and Worcestershire sauce. Add the pecans and coat with the mixture. Continue to cook over low heat for 3 to 5 minutes to roast lightly. Remove from the heat and sprinkle with cheese, tossing lightly. Spread on a cookie sheet to dry.

Exchange Values Per Tablespoon:
1 Fat

55 Calories
(87% from Fat)
1.2gm Carbohydrates
0.9gm Protein
5.5gm Fat
0.8mg Cholesterol
21mg Sodium
27mg Potassium

White Wine Melon and Cheese Appetizer

FOUR SERVINGS

1   cup cantaloupe melon balls
1   cup honeydew melon balls
⅔   cup dry white wine
3   ounces thinly sliced turkey luncheon meat, 96% fat free
7   ounces cholesterol-free white cheese, cut into ½-inch wedges
    Leaf lettuce
    Alfalfa sprouts

*C*ombine the melon balls in a small bowl and pour the wine over them. Cover and chill for 2 hours. Wrap the turkey around the cheese wedges. Drain the melon balls. Arrange the meat-cheese wedges and melon balls on a lettuce lined plate. Garnish the top with alfalfa sprouts.

Exchange Values Per Serving:
2½ Meat
½ Fruit

192 Calories
(45% from Fat)
9.3gm Carbohydrates
16.8gm Protein
9.5gm Fat
19mg Cholesterol
360mg Sodium
303mg Potassium

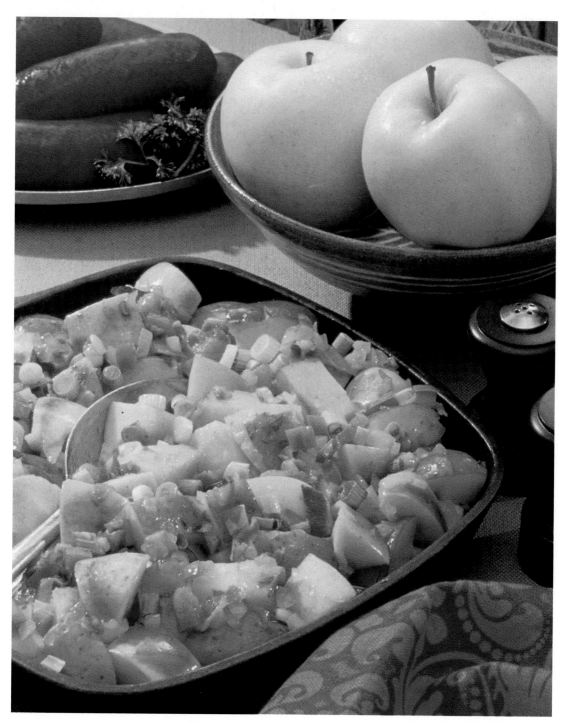

Skillet Apple Potato Salad

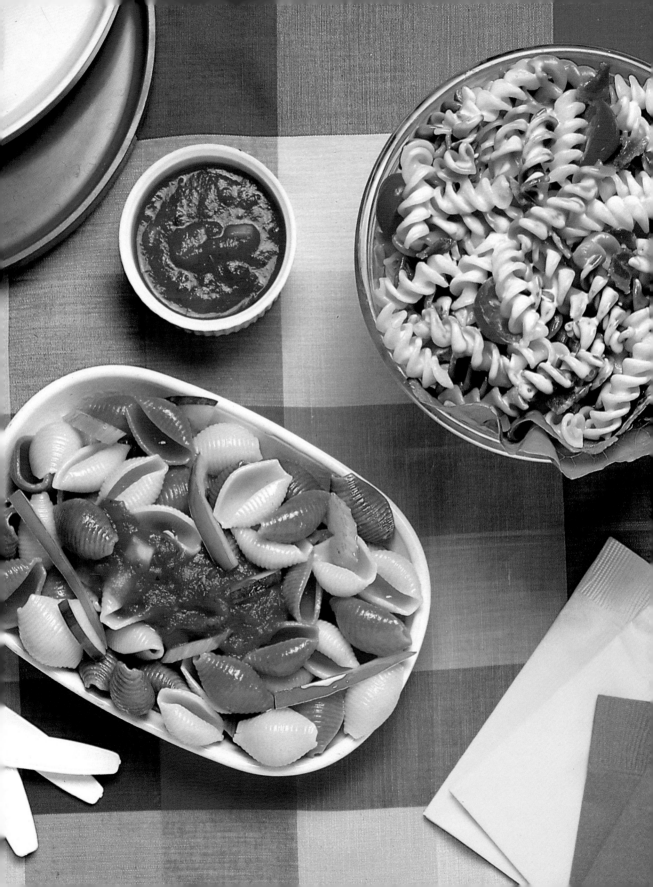

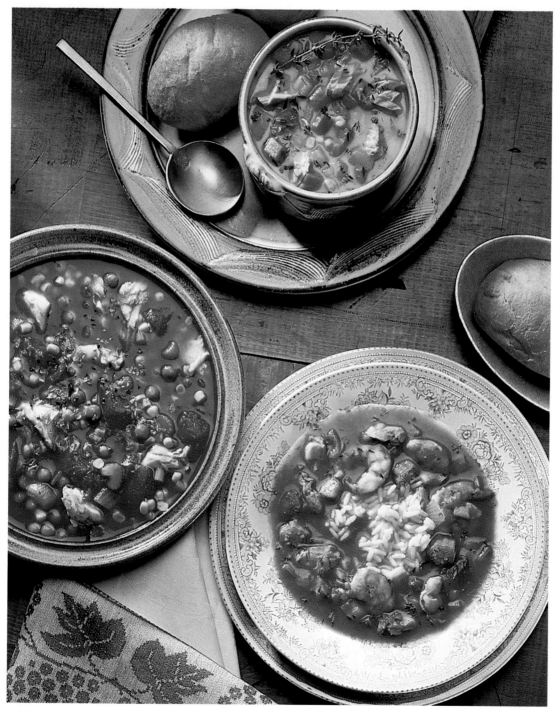

Gazpacho Salad / Pasta Salad (left)
Crab Soup / Tuna Chowder / Shrimp and Oyster Gumbo

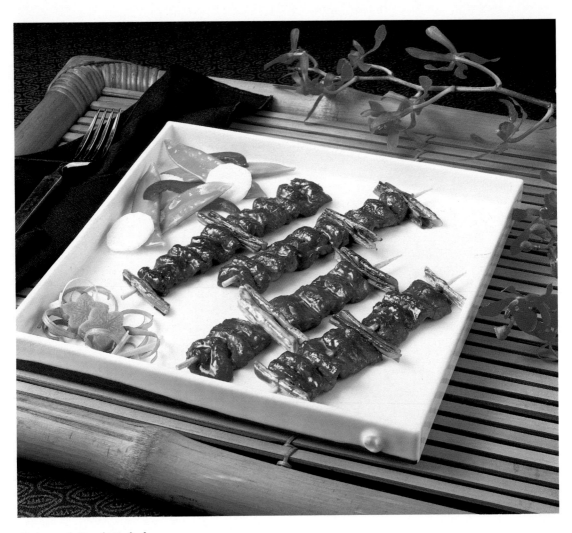

Oriental Beef Kabobs

Shrimp and Cheese Spread

TWENTY-FOUR TABLESPOONFULS

¼ cup cottage cheese
¼ cup plain lowfat yogurt
2 tablespoons tomato juice
½ teaspoon lemon juice
1 tablespoon minced parsley
1 cup ground or finely minced shrimp
¼ teaspoon paprika
   Tabasco sauce to taste

Exchange Values
Per Serving:
¼ Meat

14 Calories
(13% from Fat)
0.4gm Carbohydrates
2.3gm Protein
0.2gm Fat
14mg Cholesterol
29mg Sodium
31mg Potassium

*W*hip together the cottage cheese and yogurt to make a creamy mix. Blend in the remaining ingredients and refrigerate. Serve with crackers or celery.

Piney Cheese Ball

EIGHT SERVINGS

2 8-ounce packages Neufchatel cheese
1 8½-ounce can unsweetened crushed pineapple, drained
2 tablespoons chopped sweet onion
1 tablespoon Worcestershire sauce
1 tablespoon Beau Monde spice
1 cup chopped unsalted walnuts

Exchange Values
Per Serving:
2 Meat
2 Fat
¼ Fruit

264 Calories
(77% from Fat)
9.6gm Carbohydrates
8.1gm Protein
22.5gm Fat
42mg Cholesterol
246mg Sodium
195mg Potassium

*M*ix together all of the ingredients except the walnuts. Divide an shape into 2 balls. Chill for 30 minutes. Roll in the walnuts. This best made ahead a day or two.

Artichoke Spread

⅔ cup freshly grated Parmesan cheese
⅔ cup reduced-calorie mayonnaise
1 4½-ounce can diced green chilies
1 13½-ounce can artichoke hearts, chopped
1 teaspoon seasoned salt substitute

Combine all of the ingredients in a casserole. Microwave on high for 3 minutes or bake at 350° for 20 minutes. Serve with thinly sliced crackers.

Exchange Values
Per Tablespoon:
½ Meat
1 Fat

57 Calories
(60% from Fat)
3.6gm Carbohydrates
2.3gm Protein
3.9gm Fat
6mg Cholesterol
125mg Sodium
153mg Potassium

Oriental Beef Kabobs

10 ounces boneless beef sirloin steak, cut 1 inch thick
2   tablespoons hoisin sauce
1   tablespoon dry sherry
1   teaspoon brown sugar
½   teaspoon Oriental roasted sesame oil
3   green onions with tops, cut into 2-inch pieces

Cut the steak into ¼-inch thick strips. Combine the hoisin sauce, sherry, brown sugar, and sesame oil. Alternately weave beef strips and green onions on 8 six-inch bamboo skewers. Arrange in spoke-like fashion on a rack in a microwave-safe baking dish. Brush with the sauce. Cover with waxed paper and microwave at medium or 50 percent power for 3 minutes. Turn the kabobs over and around to bring the inside to the outside. Brush with the remaining sauce and continue cooking, covered, at medium for 2 to 3 minutes.

Exchange Values
Per Serving:
1 Meat

76 Calories
(53% from Fat)
1.5gm Carbohydrates
6.8gm Protein
4.5gm Fat
24mg Cholesterol
19mg Sodium
155mg Potassium

Holiday Chopped Liver

1 chicken or duck liver (2½ ounces)
3 tablespoons soy sauce
1 teaspoon Worcestershire sauce
1 small onion, chopped and sautéed
1 tablespoon butter, softened

*S*immer the liver in the soy and Worcestershire sauces until pink. Transfer to a food processor with the onion and pulse. Add the butter and pulse. Chill. This will stiffen as it chills.

Exchange Values Per Serving:
½ Vegetable
½ Meat
½ Fat

63 Calories
(47% from Fat)
3.5gm Carbohydrates
4.4gm Protein
3.3gm Fat
106mg Cholesterol
676mg Sodium
97mg Potassium

Sweet Meatballs

1 pound lean ground beef
¾ cup bread crumbs
1 onion, diced
¼ cup egg substitute
1 tablespoon parsley flakes
1 teaspoon pepper
1 teaspoon Worcestershire sauce

■ ■ ■

1 10¾-ounce can cream of celery soup
1 soup can skim milk

*C*ombine the ground beef, bread crumbs, onion, egg substitute, Worcestershire sauce and seasonings in a mixing bowl. Add ¼ cup of the soup to the mixture and form into meatballs. Arrange on a shallow baking sheet and bake at 350° until browned. Combine the remaining soup and skim milk in a medium saucepan to make a sauce. Add the meatballs and heat for 15 minutes.

Exchange Values Per Serving:
1 Bread
2 Meat
2 Fat

321 Calories
(52% from Fat)
17.4gm Carbohydrates
18.9gm Protein
18.9gm Fat
64mg Cholesterol
583mg Sodium
436mg Potassium

Christmas Night Miniature Meatballs

TWENTY-FOUR MEATBALLS

2 tablespoons soy sauce
¼ cup water
½ garlic clove
½ teaspoon nutmeg
1 pound lean ground chuck

Combine the soy sauce, water, minced garlic, and nutmeg in a large bowl, and stir to blend. Add the ground chuck and mix lightly but thoroughly. Form into meatballs 1 inch in diameter. Arrange in a lightly oiled baking dish. Bake uncovered at 350° for 15 minutes. Place on a heated tray or in a chafing dish and serve with toothpicks.

*Exchange Values
Per Meatball:*
½ Meat

41 Calories
(62% from Fat)
0.1gm Carbohydrates
3.7gm Protein
2.8gm Fat
12.8mg Cholesterol
76mg Sodium
48mg Potassium

Marinated Vegetables

TEN SERVINGS

1 pound asparagus
1 pound broccoli
1 pound cauliflower
1 pound baby carrots
   ■ ■ ■
12 medium mushrooms
2 cucumbers
3 tomatoes
   ■ ■ ■
1 cup virgin olive oil
1 teaspoon minced garlic
4 tablespoons dill, chopped
¼ teaspoon white pepper
2 teaspoons salt substitute

Steam the asparagus, broccoli, cauliflower, and carrots. Cool and combine with the mushrooms, cucumbers, and tomatoes. Combine the oil, garlic, dill, pepper, and salt substitute. Pour over the vegetables and chill overnight. Arrange on plates for a beautiful luncheon start.

*Exchange Values
Per Serving:*
3 Vegetable
2 Fat

162 Calories
(63% from Fat)
14.2gm Carbohydrates
4.2gm Protein
11.4gm Fat
0mg Cholesterol
43mg Sodium
1236mg Potassium

Italian Carrot Antipasto

SIX SERVINGS

1 pound tender young carrots
¾ cup dry white wine
¾ cup white wine vinegar
4 cups water
6 tablespoons oil
2 cloves garlic
  Small bunch parsley
1 teaspoon celery seeds
1 teaspoon sugar
  Pinch pepper

■ ■ ■

1 teaspoon chopped basil
1 teaspoon spicy mustard
1 head of lettuce, chopped

Exchange Values
Per Serving:
2 Vegetable
3 Fat

193 Calories
(66% from Fat)
13.9gm Carbohydrates
1.9gm Protein
14.1gm Fat
0mg Cholesterol
49mg Sodium
434mg Potassium

*W*ash and scrape the carrots, and cut them into strips. Combine the carrots, wine, vinegar, water, oil, garlic, parsley, celery seed, sugar, and pepper in an enamel saucepan. Bring to a boil over moderate heat and cook for about 10 minutes. Remove from the heat and allow to cool.

Remove the carrots and boil the marinade until reduced to about 2 cups. Toss the carrots with the chopped lettuce. Place in a serving dish. Pour the marinade over them and sprinkle with basil. Toss with the mustard and chill.

Your Own Crispy Crackers

NINETEEN SERVINGS

2 cups rolled oats, quick-cooking or regular
1½ cups all-purpose flour
⅓ cup finely ground pecans
1½ tablespoons brown sugar
1 teaspoon salt substitute
⅔ cup water
½ cup safflower oil
6 tablespoons sesame seeds

Exchange Values
Per 5 Crackers:
1 Bread
2 Fat

*C*rush the oats in a food processor. Combine the crushed oats, flour, pecans, brown sugar, and salt substitute in a large bowl. Mix until well blended. Add the water and oil, and blend thoroughly. Divide dough into 3 balls. Place each ball on a 16x12-inch baking sheet. Roll the dough all the way to the edges; this will be very thin. Sprinkle the dough lightly with sesame seeds. With a pastry wheel or pizza wheel, cut the dough into 2-inch squares or diamonds. Bake at 325° for 30 to 35 minutes or until golden brown. Remove carefully with a spatula. Store in an airtight container for up to a month. These may also be frozen.

160 Calories
(58% from Fat)
14gm Carbohydrates
3.0gm Protein
10.0gm Fat
0mg Cholesterol
9mg Sodium
39mg Potassium

Stuffed Dill Mushrooms

EIGHTEEN MUSHROOMS

24 **large mushrooms**
3 **scallions, cut into 2-inch pieces**
3 **tablespoons liquid margarine**
⅛ **teaspoon white pepper**
¾ **ounce grated Parmesan cheese**
2 **tablespoons diced dill weed**
6 **ounces lowfat cottage cheese**

Exchange Values
Per Mushroom:
1 Fat

41 Calories
(46% from Fat)
2.3gm Carbohydrates
2.7gm Protein
2.6gm Fat
2mg Cholesterol
81mg Sodium
158mg Potassium

*R*emove the stems from 18 of the mushrooms, reserve. Cut the remaining mushrooms in quarters, and finely chop with the metal blade in a food processor for 25 pulses. Set aside. Finely chop the scallions, and set aside. Sauté the chopped mushrooms in melted margarine until done, about 4 minutes. Add the scallions and cook for 30 seconds to wilt. Season with pepper, and reserve. With the metal blade of a food processor, process the Parmesan and dill until fine. Add the cottage cheese and process until smooth. Add the mushroom and scallion mixture and pulse 5 times. Cover and chill until firm, about 30 minutes.

Fill each mushroom cap with the mushroom and cheese mixture and place on a greased cookie sheet. Broil at 400° for about 4 minutes, until slightly bubbly, then reduce the temperature to 300° and cook for 4 to 5 minutes more. The mushrooms should be firm. Serve immediately.

Broiled Stuffed Mushrooms

FIVE SERVINGS

20 large mushrooms with stems, cleaned and dry
1 tablespoon liquid margarine
1 scallion, minced
¼ cup lowfat cottage cheese
1 tablespoon chopped fresh parsley
1 small tomato, peeled, seeded and chopped
½ teaspoon Worcestershire sauce
3 tablespoons Parmesan cheese

Exchange Values
Per 4 Mushrooms:
1 Vegetable
1 Fat

80 Calories
(49% from Fat)
5.6gm Carbohydrates
5.6gm Protein
4.4gm Fat
4.8mg Cholesterol
176mg Sodium
380mg Potassium

Remove the stems from the mushrooms and chop the stems finely. Melt the margarine in a skillet and sauté the scallion and mushroom stems. When most of the liquid is gone, remove from the heat and cool. Place the cottage cheese, parsley, tomato, and Worcestershire sauce in a food processor. Pulsate. Add the stems and scallions, and stir until well blended. Stuff the caps with the creamy mixture. Place on a cookie sheet. Sprinkle with Parmesan cheese and broil until slightly brown.

Cheddar-Dijon Dip

TEN SERVINGS

2 cups shredded imitation sharp Cheddar cheese
2 tablespoons liquid margarine
1 tablespoon Dijon mustard
1 8-ounce container plain lowfat yogurt
½ cup chopped pecans
2 tablespoons chopped parsley

Exchange Values
Per Serving:
1 Fat
2 Meat

148 Calories
(70% from Fat)
4.5gm Carbohydrates
7.7gm Protein
11.6gm Fat
1.7mg Cholesterol
410mg Sodium
116mg Potassium

Process the cheese, margarine, and mustard in a blender container or food processor bowl with a metal blade, until smooth. Add the yogurt and blend until smooth. Spoon the mixture into a bowl and gently stir in the pecans and parsley. Refrigerate for 1 to 2 hours. Serve as a dip with vegetables or crackers. One serving equals 3 tablespoons.

Dilly Dip

SIXTEEN TABLESPOONFULS

¾ cup plain lowfat yogurt
⅓ cup lite mayonnaise
1 tablespoon instant minced onion
1 teaspoon celery salt
1 tablespoon parsley flakes
1 tablespoon dill weed

*C*ombine all of the ingredients in a small bowl, and mix well. Cover and refrigerate for several hours to blend the flavors. Serve with raw vegetables.

Exchange Values Per Tablespoon:
½ Fat

20 Calories
(66% from Fat)
1.2gm Carbohydrates
0.6gm Protein
1.5gm Fat
2.3mg Cholesterol
136mg Sodium
25mg Potassium

Guacamole Dip

TWENTY-FOUR TABLESPOONFULS

2 large avocados, pitted and peeled
2 tablespoons of plain lowfat yogurt
⅛ teaspoon garlic powder
1 teaspoon lemon or lime juice
½ can chopped green chilies (about ⅓ cup)
　 Tabasco sauce to taste
½ small onion, chopped
1 small tomato, chopped

*M*ash the avocado in a food processor. Add the yogurt, garlic powder, lemon or lime juice, green chilies, Tabasco, onion, and tomato. Puree in the processor until smooth. Refrigerate. This dip is best if refrigerated for 2 days to allow the flavors to blend. One serving equals about 1½ tablespoonfuls.

Exchange Values Per Serving:
1 Fat

43 Calories
(81% from Fat)
2.4gm Carbohydrates
0.6gm Protein
3.9gm Fat
0.2mg Cholesterol
50mg Sodium
175mg Potassium

Mexican Salsa

SIXTEEN TABLESPOONFULS

2   medium tomatoes
2   garlic cloves, crushed
⅓ cup chopped onion
1   teaspoon Worcestershire sauce
⅓ to ½ green chilie salsa
2   tablespoons salsa jalapena

*P*lace whole tomatoes in a small shallow pan. Broil under medium heat. Turn the tomatoes on all sides until the skins are blistered and burnt and the tomatoes are cooked through, 10 to 15 minutes. Cool. Place the tomatoes in a blender or food processor fitted with the metal blade. Add the remaining ingredients and mix until blended. Refrigerate for several hours before serving. This may be stored in the refrigerator for several months. Up to 3 tablespoonfuls several times a day is allowed.

Exchange Values Per Tablespoon:
Free

5 Calories
(0% from Fat)
5.6gm Carbohydrates
0.2gm Protein
0gm Fat
0mg Cholesterol
147mg Sodium
229mg Potassium

Hotty Totty Onion Dip

FORTY-EIGHT TABLESPOONFULS

1   10½-ounce can low-sodium condensed cream of onion soup
1   cup (8 ounces) plain lowfat yogurt
1   cup (8 ounces) reduced sodium salsa

*C*ombine all of the ingredients in a medium saucepan. Cover and cook slowly to warm throughout. Serve warm with vegetables. 2 tablespoonfuls several times a day is allowed.

Exchange Values Per Tablespoon:
Free

9 Calories
(44% from Fat)
1gm Carbohydrates
0.4gm Protein
0.5gm Fat
0.3mg Cholesterol
65mg Sodium
26mg Potassium

Munchy Crunchy Vegetable Dip

FIFTY-SIX TABLESPOONFULS

1½ cups plain lowfat yogurt
1   cup lite mayonnaise
1   8-ounce can water chestnuts, drained, finely chopped
½ cup finely chopped carrots
½ cup finely chopped broccoli
1   package low sodium dry vegetable soup mix
1   teaspoon Worcestershire sauce

Combine all the ingredients in a medium bowl and mix well. Cover and refrigerate for several hours to allow the flavors to blend. Serve with vegetables.

Exchange Values Per Tablespoon:
½ Fat

19 Calories
(42% from Fat)
1.3gm Carbohydrates
0.4gm Protein
1.4gm Fat
3.8mg Cholesterol
31mg Sodium
35mg Potassium

Spinach Vegetable Dip

FIFTY-SIX TABLESPOONFULS

1   8-ounce container plain lowfat yogurt
1   cup reduced-calorie mayonnaise
¾ package low sodium dry leek soup mix
1   10-ounce package frozen chopped spinach, well drained
½ cup chopped parsley
½ cup chopped green onions
1   teaspoon dry dill
1   teaspoon dry Italian salad dressing mix

In a food processor combine all of the ingredients and mix until well incorporated. Place in an airtight container and refrigerate. Just before serving, place in a bowl and surround with raw vegetables.

Exchange Values Per Tablespoon:
1 Fat

49 Calories
(45% from Fat)
6.1gm Carbohydrates
1.9gm Protein
2.9gm Fat
3.4mg Cholesterol
273mg Sodium
141mg Potassium

Hot Spiced Tea

2   3-ounce packages sugar-free strawberry gelatin
½   gallon boiling water

   ■ ■ ■

6   cinnamon sticks
12 cloves
1   pint water
1   quart weak tea
1   cup pure lemon juice
1   quart of water
8   packets artificial sweetener or to taste
1   46-ounce can pineapple juice, unsweetened

*Exchange Values
Per Serving:*
½ Fruit

31 Calories
(0% from Fat)
5gm Carbohydrates
4.1gm Protein
0gm Fat
0mg Cholesterol
9mg Sodium
37mg Potassium

*D*issolve the gelatin in boiling water. In a separate pan, simmer the cinnamon sticks and cloves in 1 pint of water for 30 minutes. Combine all of the ingredients. Add more water or juice if desired. Serve warm but do not boil. One serving equals 6 ounces.

Chocolate Cafe Borgia

TWELVE SERVINGS

1   12-pack box instant sugar-free hot cocoa mix
12 cups of freshly perked coffee
    Whipped cream
    Grated orange peel

*I*n a large mug combine 1 packet of the cocoa mix with 1 cup of hot coffee. Stir well. Garnish each 6-ounce serving with 2 tablespoons whipped cream and sprinkle with grated orange peel.

Exchange Values
Per Serving:
1 Milk

89 Calories
(42% from Fat)
10.0gm Carbohydrates
4.4gm Protein
4.2gm Fat
13.0mg Cholesterol
192mg Sodium
551mg Potassium

Christmas Wassail

TWENTY SERVINGS

4   cups unsweetened apple juice
3   cups low-calorie unsweetened pineapple juice
2   cups cranberry juice cocktail
¼   teaspoon ground nutmeg
1   cinnamon stick, broken in half
2   whole cloves

    ▪ ▪ ▪

4   packets artificial sweetener
    Lemon slices
    Apple slices
    Orange slices

*C*ombine the apple juice, pineapple juice, cranberry juice, nutmeg, cinnamon stick, and cloves. Simmer for 10 minutes; do not boil. Pour into a punch bowl and add the sweetener, lemon slices, apple slices, and orange slices to the top. Stir and serve.

Exchange Values
Per Serving:
1 Fruit

60 Calories
(2% from Fat)
15gm Carbohydrates
0.2gm Protein
0.1gm Fat
0mg Cholesterol
3mg Sodium
119mg Potassium

Fall Apple Coffee

EIGHT SERVINGS

1 quart unsweetened apple juice
1 quart hot, strong black coffee
6 oranges, sliced wafer thin
2 3-inch cinnamon sticks
  Pinch allspice
  Pinch nutmeg
  Pinch cloves
  Brown sugar substitute to equal ⅓ cup brown sugar

Exchange Values Per Serving:
2 Fruit

109 Calories
(2% from Fat)
26.5gm Carbohydrates
1gm Protein
1gm Fat
0mg Cholesterol
8mg Sodium
394mg Potassium

*P*lace all of the ingredients except the brown sugar substitute in a large saucepan and bring to a boil over medium heat. Reduce heat and simmer for 10 minutes. Remove from the heat and add the brown sugar substitute. Stir well and pour into a pitcher. Serve in 8-ounce mugs.

Hot Spiced Coffee

FOUR SERVINGS

3 cups strong hot coffee
1 cinnamon stick
3 whole cloves
½ teaspoon ground allspice
1 tablespoon grated orange rinds
  Artificial sweetener to taste

Exchange Values Per Serving:
Free

7 Calories
(0% from Fat)
0.8gm Carbohydrates
0gm Protein
0gm Fat
0mg Cholesterol
7mg Sodium
103mg Potassium

*P*our the coffee into a pitcher and stir in the cinnamon stick, cloves, allspice, and orange rinds. Let stand for 2 hours. Pour the coffee through a sieve to remove the cloves and cinnamon sticks. Pour into tall glasses filled with ice and add artificial sweetener to taste. Garnish with an orange wedge.

Instant Breakfast Drink

THIRTY-TWO SERVINGS

2 cups orange sugar-free instant breakfast drink
1 cup unsweetened instant tea mix
1 teaspoon ground cloves
1 teaspoon ground cinnamon

*C*ombine all of the ingredients and mix well. Store in an airtight container. To serve, put 2 rounded tablespoons of mix in each cup. Fill with boiling water and stir well.

Exchange Values Per Serving:
Free

3 Calories
(0% from Fat)
0.7gm Carbohydrates
0gm Protein
0gm Fat
0mg Cholesterol
0mg Sodium
70mg Potassium

Orange Monster Drink

SIXTEEN SERVINGS

2 quarts fresh, unsweetened orange juice
3 3-inch cinnamon sticks
20 whole cloves
3 tablespoons grated orange peel
8 packets artificial sweetener

*P*lace all of the ingredients except the sweetener in a large saucepan. Bring to a boil, reduce the heat, and simmer for 5 minutes. Strain the grog through a colander or sieve into a large pitcher and add the sweetener. Pour into 4-ounce mugs.

Exchange Values Per Serving:
1 Fruit

56 Calories
(4% from Fat)
12.9gm Carbohydrates
0.9gm Protein
0.3gm Fat
0mg Cholesterol
1mg Sodium
248mg Potassium

A Peach of a Punch

FOURTEEN SERVINGS

1 46-ounce can unsweetened pure peach nectar
4 peaches, cored, peeled and pureed
2 cups fresh orange juice

■ ■ ■

3 2-inch cinnamon sticks, crumbled
6 whole cloves
1 teaspoon nutmeg
2 tablespoons lime juice, fresh if possible
¼ cup brown sugar substitute

Exchange Values
Per Serving:
1½ Fruit

84 Calories
(1% from Fat)
21.4gm Carbohydrates
0.7gm Protein
0.1gm Fat
0mg Cholesterol
7mg Sodium
163mg Potassium

Combine the peach nectar, pureed peaches, and orange juice in a large saucepan. Bring to a boil, reduce the heat, and simmer. Add the spices and stir. Add the lime juice and stir. Remove from the heat and add the brown sugar substitute. Stir until well blended and dissolved. Place a strainer over a prewarmed punch bowl and strain the punch into it. Ladle into 5-ounce punch cups and sprinkle each with a bit of grated orange peel.

Spiced Russian Tea

EIGHTEEN SERVINGS

2 quarts water
1 cinnamon stick, broken in half
10 whole cloves
6 tea bags

■ ■ ■

Juice of 2 oranges
Juice of 1 lemon
¼ cup cranapple juice
4 packets sugar substitute

Exchange Values
Per Serving:
Free

6 Calories
(3% from Fat)
1.5gm Carbohydrates
0.1gm Protein
0gm Fat
0mg Cholesterol
5mg Sodium
35mg Potassium

Bring the water to a boil with the cinnamon stick and cloves. Reduce the heat to a simmer and add the tea bags. Brew until a deep golden tea. Strain the tea through a cloth. Pour into a 4-quart container and add the juices and artificial sweetener. Serve warm or over ice in 4-ounce cups.

Warmed Wintery Milk

THREE SERVINGS

3 cups skim milk
2 packets of artificial sweetener
½ teaspoon almond extract
1 teaspoon rum flavoring

*I*n a small saucepan, warm the milk to scald only. Remove from the heat and add the sweetener and flavorings. Stir to blend well. Serve immediately in warmed mugs or pour into a thermos for travel in cold weather.

Exchange Values Per Serving:
1 Milk

90 Calories
(5% from Fat)
11.9gm Carbohydrates
8.3gm Protein
0.3gm Fat
3mg Cholesterol
130mg Sodium
408mg Potassium

Creamed Iced Tea

SIX SERVINGS

6 tea bags
3 cups boiling water
1 28-ounce bottle sugar-free cream soda

*S*teep the tea bags in boiling water for 3 to 5 minutes. Pour the tea into a large pitcher. When ready to serve add the cream soda. Serve in 8-ounce glasses over ice and garnish with fruit.

Exchange Values Per Serving:
Free

0 Calories
(0% from Fat)
0gm Carbohydrates
0gm Protein
0gm Fat
0mg Cholesterol
39mg Sodium
31mg Potassium

Chocolate-Coffee Milkshake

1 cup cold skim milk
3 ice cubes, crushed
1 teaspoon instant coffee
1 teaspoon instant sugar-free cocoa mix
  Artificial sweetener to taste

*P*lace all of the ingredients in a blender and blend until creamy.
Serve over ice.

Exchange Values
Per Serving:
½ Milk

56 Calories
(5% from Fat)
7.3gm Carbohydrates
4.9gm Protein
0.3gm Fat
2mg Cholesterol
98mg Sodium
227mg Potassium

Tea Punch

6 cups extra strong tea
3 cups unsweetened orange juice
2 cups unsweetened grapefruit juice
½ cup lime juice
½ cup lemon juice

■ ■ ■

2 28-ounce bottles sugar-free ginger ale
  Mint sprigs and wafer-thin lemon slices to float
  Artificial sweetener to taste

*C*ombine the tea and the juices in a punch bowl and stir well. Refrigerate until ready to serve.
    Just before serving, add sugar-free ginger ale and some ice cubes
or ice fruit cubes and stir. Garnish the punch with mint sprigs and
lemon slices. Have artificial sweetener available for those that want
it a little sweeter. One serving equals 4 ounces.

Exchange Values
Per Serving:
⅓ Fruit

14 Calories
(2% from Fat)
3.5gm Carbohydrates
0.2gm Protein
0.1gm Fat
0mg Cholesterol
7mg Sodium
73mg Potassium

Mint Tea

SIX SERVINGS

2 cups green mint, slashed or chopped
2 lemons
1 quart water
6 packets artificial sweetener
1 quart unsweetened tea
6 fresh cherries

*P*lace the chopped mint in a large stew pot. Peel the lemons and shred the rind. Sprinkle over the mint. Place the water in the stew pan and add the juice of both lemons. Bring to a boil and turn off the heat immediately. Remove from the heat and pour over the mint and lemon rinds. Cover the mint mixture and let it stand until cool. When cool use a potato masher to press more mint into the juice. Strain off the juice. Add the sweetener. This will make 1 quart. Refrigerate.

Add to an unsweetened tea in equal parts as needed. Serve with a fresh cherry and a sprig of mint.

Exchange Values
Per Serving:
Free

16 Calories
(0% from Fat)
3.3gm Carbohydrates
0.3gm Protein
0gm Fat
10mg Cholesterol
102mg Sodium

Southern Mint Juleps

TEN SERVINGS

4 or 5 sprigs of fresh mint
2 cups cold water
¾ cup lemon juice (fresh, if possible)
1½ quarts sugar-free ginger ale
10 packets artificial sweetener

*R*inse the mint leaves and discard the stems. Place the water and lemon juice in a medium size pitcher and mix. Stir in the mint leaves and the artificial sweetener. Let stand for 30 minutes. Fill a large pitcher with ice cubes, and strain the liquid over the ice. Add the ginger ale and float lemon slices on the top of the drinks.

Exchange Values
Per Serving:
Free

9 Calories
(0% from Fat)
2.6gm Carbohydrates
0.1gm Protein
0gm Fat
0mg Cholesterol
31mg Sodium
25mg Potassium

An Apricot Drink

3 cups chopped fresh apricots, skins removed, or drained canned
  apricots
4 tablespoons unsweetened 100% fruit apricot preserves
4 cups plain lowfat yogurt
  Skim milk as needed to make a smooth drink

*P*lace the apricots and preserves in a food processor or blender and
process until pureed, about 2 minutes. Add the yogurt and pulse
again to blend. Add just enough milk to make a creamy consistency.
Refrigerate for 1 hour. One serving equals 10 ounces.

*Exchange Values
Per Serving:*
1 Fruit
1 Milk

160 Calories
(16% from Fat)
26.6gm Carbohydrates
9.5gm Protein
2.6gm Fat
9.7mg Cholesterol
120mg Sodium
620mg Potassium

Blackberry Buzz

1 cup lemonade, artificially sweetened and made from a
  concentrate
2 cups canned or frozen blackberries, with juice
1 cup club soda

■ ■ ■

1 quart sugar-free ginger ale

*C*ombine all of the ingredients except the ginger ale in a blender and
blend for 20 seconds or until smooth. Put some ice cubes in frosted
tankards, and add 4 ounces of the blender mixture until they are half
filled. Fill the tankards with ginger ale, stir, and serve. Artificial
sweetener may be needed to sweeten to taste.

*Exchange Values
Per Serving:*
½ Fruit

27 Calories
(5% from Fat)
6.5gm Carbohydrates
0.3gm Protein
0.1gm Fat
0mg Cholesterol
31mg Sodium
83mg Potassium

Brunch Punch

FORTY SERVINGS

1 cup fresh unsweetened orange juice
1 cup lemonade, artificially sweetened
1 cup limeade
1 cup tangerine juice, or 2 tangerines sqeezed to make 1 cup of
   juice
1 46-ounce can pineapple juice unsweetened

■ ■ ■

2 quarts chilled sugar-free ginger ale

*P*lace all of the ingredients except the ginger ale in a large pitcher and blend well. Chill 2 hours. When ready to serve, place in a punch bowl and add the ginger ale. One serving equals 3½ ounces.

Exchange Values Per Serving:
½ Fruit

26 Calories
(2% from Fat)
6.4gm Carbohydrates
0.2gm Protein
0.1gm Fat
0mg Cholesterol
11mg Sodium
70mg Potassium

Cantaloupe Refresher

SIX SERVINGS

1 medium ripe cantaloupe, diced
3 tablespoons lime juice
2 cups orange juice
2 packets artificial sweetener
½ cup diabetic vanilla ice cream

*P*lace all of the ingredients except the ice cream in a blender and blend until smooth. Add the ice cream and puree. One serving equals 5 ounces.

Exchange Values Per Serving:
1 Fruit
½ Fat

91 Calories
(16% from Fat)
18.8gm Carbohydrates
1.6gm Protein
1.5gm Fat
0mg Cholesterol
5mg Sodium
336mg Potassium

Citrus Punch

TWELVE SERVINGS

6   small tea bags
4   cups boiling water
8   packets artificial sweetener
1   6-ounce can frozen orange juice, thawed and undiluted
1   6-ounce can frozen lemonade, thawed and undiluted
10 cups cold water

*S*teep the tea bags in boiling water for about 5 minutes. Do not boil. Discard the tea bags and add the remaining ingredients. Serve over ice. One serving equals 5 ounces.

Exchange Values Per Serving:
1 Fruit

51 Calories
(1% from Fat)
12.2gm Carbohydrates
0.6gm Protein
0gm Fat
0mg Cholesterol
5mg Sodium
191mg Potassium

Cranberry Fizz Punch

TWENTY-SIX SERVINGS

1   6-ounce can frozen lemonade concentrate, unsweetened
1   quart low-calorie cranberry juice
1   30-ounce can unsweetened pineapple juice
1   6-ounce can unsweetened frozen orange juice concentrate

1   quart sugar-free ginger ale, chilled

*R*econstitute the lemonade and orange juice according to the package directions. Pour into a large container. Add the cranberry and pineapple juices. Chill. Add the ginger ale just before serving. One serving equals 5 ounces.

Exchange Values Per Serving:
1 Fruit

59 Calories
(1% from Fat)
15.0gm Carbohydrates
0.3gm Protein
0.1gm Fat
0mg Cholesterol
11mg Sodium
110mg Potassium

Frosty Strawberry Delight

FOUR SERVINGS

2½ cups fresh ripe strawberries
1   8-ounce container plain lowfat yogurt
1   cup skim milk
½   cup sugar-free red pop
2   packages artificial sweetener

In a blender or food processor mix the strawberries, yogurt, and skim milk. Slowly stir in the red pop and serve. Garnish with a whole strawberry and mint leaf.

Exchange Values
Per Serving:
1 Milk
1 Fruit

144 Calories
(15% from Fat)
25.1gm Carbohydrates
11.0gm Protein
2.3gm Fat
4mg Cholesterol
165mg Sodium
330mg Potassium

Fruit Cubes and Fizz

TWO SERVINGS

2½ cups strawberries, halved
¼   cup lemon juice

■ ■ ■

Sugar-free red soda or lemon-lime soda

In a small narrow bowl, dip each strawberry into the lemon juice and place on a cookie sheet so that the fruit is not touching. Place in the freezer and allow to freeze solid. When frozen these pieces can be transferred to a freezer bag and kept until needed.

Place half of the strawberries in a glass and fill with soda. A great drink, pretty to look at, the frozen fruit won't dilute the drink.

Exchange Values
Per Serving:
1 Fruit

63 Calories
(11% from Fat)
15.2gm Carbohydrates
1.3gm Protein
0.8gm Fat
0mg Cholesterol
26mg Sodium
343mg Potassium

Fruity Good Morning Drink

1   banana
1   cup plain lowfat yogurt
1   cup unsweetened orange juice, chilled
1¼ cups hulled strawberries
½   teaspoon vanilla extract
1   packet artificial sweetener

■ ■ ■

3   fresh mint sprigs

*B*lend all of the ingredients except the mint in a blender. Pour into 4 5-ounce glasses. Garnish with fresh mint.

Exchange Values Per Serving:
½ Milk
1 Fruit

106 Calories
(11% from Fat)
20.5gm Carbohydrates
3.9gm Protein
1.3gm Fat
3mg Cholesterol
55mg Sodium
436mg Potassium

A Fruity Punch

1   3-ounce box sugar-free cherry gelatin
1   quart boiling water
3   quarts cool water
1   46-ounce can pineapple juice, unsweetened

■ ■ ■

1   quart sugar-free lemon-lime soda

*D*issolve the gelatin in the boiling water. Add the cool water and pineapple juice. Chill in the refrigerator. When ready to serve, pour into a punch bowl and add the sugar-free soda. Stir well. Garnish with sliced lemons and limes. One serving equals 4 ounces.

This is a beautiful punch for weddings and at Christmas.

Exchange Values Per Serving:
¼ Fruit

22 Calories
(1% from Fat)
3.6gm Carbohydrates
1.3gm Protein
0.1gm Fat
0mg Cholesterol
6mg Sodium
39mg Potassium

A Fruit Shake

FOUR SERVINGS

1 cup vanilla lowfat yogurt
½ cup sliced fresh strawberries
½ cup diced fresh papaya
½ cup diced ripe cantaloupe
4 packets artificial sweetener
1 cup crushed ice
½ cup extra cantaloupe for garnish

*P*lace the yogurt, strawberries, papaya, cantaloupe, and sweetener in a food processor or blender. Process until smooth. Add the crushed ice and blend thoroughly again. Pour into frosted glasses and garnish with cantaloupe slices.

*Exchange Values
Per Serving:*
1 Fruit

60 Calories
(15% from Fat)
9.7gm Carbohydrates
3.4gm Protein
1gm Fat
3.5mg Cholesterol
42mg Sodium
357mg Potassium

Fruity Slush

TWENTY-FIVE SERVINGS

6 packets artificial sweetener
6 cups water
1 46-ounce can unsweetened pineapple juice
2 12-ounce cans unsweetened frozen orange juice, undiluted
1 12-ounce can unsweetened frozen lemonade, undiluted
5 bananas

■ ■ ■

Sugar-free lemon lime soft drink

*B*ring the water to a boil, cool for 10 minutes, and then stir in the sugar substitute. Add the remaining ingredients except the lemon lime drink and pour into 5 1-quart freezer containers or several ice cube trays. Freeze.

When ready to serve, fill glasses half full of lemon-lime flavored soft drink, 5 ounces of the mixture, and several ice cubes. Serve with a sprig of mint and a colorful straw.

*Exchange Values
Per Serving:*
2 Fruit

120 Calories
(2% from Fat)
29.6gm Carbohydrates
1.2gm Protein
0.2gm Fat
0mg Cholesterol
21mg Sodium
359mg Potassium

Lime and Raspberry Refresher

1 cup crushed frozen or fresh unsweetened raspberries
⅓ cup lime juice (about 4 fresh limes, squeezed)
1½ quarts sugar-free ginger ale
Artificial sweetener to taste if needed

*I*n a food processor, process the raspberries and lime juice. Carefully stir in the ginger ale and serve over crushed ice. Add sweetener if needed.

Exchange Values Per Serving:
⅓ Fruit

21 Calories
(8% from Fat)
5.3gm Carbohydrates
0.2gm Protein
0.2gm Fat
0mg Cholesterol
60mg Sodium
69mg Potassium

Orange Frosty

1 6-ounce can 100% unsweetened orange juice concentrate, undiluted
2 cups skim milk
1 teaspoon vanilla extract
2 packages artificial sweetener
½ cup crushed ice

*C*ombine all of the ingredients in a food processor and blend until smooth. Serve immediately. One serving equals 11 ounces.

Exchange Values Per Serving:
½ Milk
1 Fruit

116 Calories
(2% from Fat)
22.5gm Carbohydrates
5.2gm Protein
0.4gm Fat
2.7mg Cholesterol
69mg Sodium
491mg Potassium

Strawberry Grog

1 2-liter container sugar-free lemon-lime or club soda
1 .6-ounce package sugar-free strawberry gelatin
  Crushed ice

*C*arefully pour the gelatin into the soft drink and cap immediately. Place this in the refrigerator until morning. Serve over crushed ice.

Exchange Values Per Serving:
Free

5 Calories
(0% from Fat)
0gm Carbohydrates
0.9gm Protein
0gm Fat
0mg Cholesterol
40mg Sodium
31mg Potassium

Strawberry Parfait Drink

1 pint fresh strawberries, cleaned and choped (or 2 cups frozen)
½ cup skim evaporated milk
½ cup vanilla lowfat yogurt
2 cups ice, crushed
2 packets artificial sweetener
6 whole strawberries for garnish

*C*ombine all of the ingredients except the strawberries for the garnish in a blender. Blend at high speed until smooth. Serve in punch cups or in tulip champagne glasses, with a strawberry on the side of the glass. One serving equals 6 ounces.

Exchange Values Per Serving:
½ Milk
½ Fruit

53 Calories
(10% from Fat)
9.6gm Carbohydrates
2.9gm Protein
0.5gm Fat
2.0mg Cholesterol
38mg Sodium
197mg Potassium

Tart and Bubbly Wake-Up Drink

TWO SERVINGS

½ cup unsweetened pineapple juice
3 cranberry-raspberry ice cubes
½ cup sugar-free lemon-lime soda

*C*ombine all of the ingredients in a pitcher and serve in 2 chilled wine glasses.

In the place of pineapple juice, you can substitute orange juice or apple juice. Sugar-free red pop also adds a twist to this drink.

Exchange Values Per Serving:
1 Fruit

55 Calories
(1% from Fat)
14gm Carbohydrates
0.2gm Protein
0.1gm Fat
0mg Cholesterol
15mg Sodium
93mg Potassium

Breakfast Tomato Juice

ONE SERVING

1 6-ounce can tomato juice
½ teaspoon lemon juice
   Dash Worcestershire sauce
   Dash salt
1 packet artificial sweetener

*C*ombine all of the ingredients in a glass. Stir to blend.

Exchange Values Per Serving:
1½ Vegetable

40 Calories
(2% from Fat)
9.8gm Carbohydrates
1.5gm Protein
0.1gm Fat
0mg Cholesterol
768mg Sodium
622mg Potassium

A Carrot Cocktail

SIX SERVINGS

3 cups unsweetened pineapple juice
2 large carrots, cut into very small pieces
½ teaspoon lemon juice
¼ cup plain lowfat yogurt
1 cup crushed ice

*P*lace the pineapple juice and carrots in a food processor or blender and liquify. Add the remaining ingredients and blend again until liquified. Serve immediately. One serving equals 5 ounces.

Exchange Values Per Serving:
1 Fruit

86 Calories
(3% from Fat)
20.3gm Carbohydrates
1.1gm Protein
0.3gm Fat
0.6mg Cholesterol
16mg Sodium
267mg Potassium

Tomato and Celery Curry Drink

SIX SERVINGS

1 46-ounce can tomato juice
1 teaspoon curry powder
½ cup celery juice (purchased or strained from pureed celery)
  Dash Tabasco

*P*lace ½ cup of the tomato juice in a small bowl, add the curry powder and stir to blend well. Add the celery juice, Tabasco and remaining tomato juice, and heat to boiling. Refrigerate. Pour chilled juice into a thermos or serve in mugs. One serving equals 8 ounces.

Exchange Values Per Serving:
2 Vegetable

43 Calories
(3% from Fat)
10.7gm Carbohydrates
2gm Protein
0.2gm Fat
0mg Cholesterol
821mg Sodium
790mg Potassium

Hearty Tomato Saucy Drink

TWO SERVINGS

10 ounces stewed tomatoes, fresh or canned
2 tablespoons lemon juice
2 tablespoons lime juice
1 teaspoon Worcestershire sauce
4 drops Tabasco
1 cup cold water

*P*lace the stewed tomatoes, juices, and seasonings in a blender and blend for 30 seconds on medium speed. Add the cold water, stir, and pour into old-fashioned glasses filled with crushed ice. Garnish each with a slice of lime.

Exchange Values Per Serving:
1 Vegetable

44 Calories
(10% from Fat)
10.5gm Carbohydrates
1.7gm Protein
0.5gm Fat
0mg Cholesterol
48mg Sodium
416mg Potassium

Tomato Frappe

SIX SERVINGS

1 tablespoon liquid margarine
3 tablespoons finely chopped onion
1 tablespoon lemon juice
   Generous dash of Worcestershire sauce
   Generous dash of Tabasco sauce
4 cups pure tomato juice

*M*elt the margarine and sauté the chopped onion until tender and translucent. Place the sautéed onion, lemon juice, Worcestershire, and Tabasco in a blender. Blend for 1 minute or until smooth. Pour into a metal baking pan and freeze. Half an hour before needed, take the tomato mix out of the freezer. Allow to thaw just enough to break into chunks. Place in a food processor and blend until smooth. Don't let it melt. Serve in sherbet glasses with a lemon wedge and straws. One serving equals 5 ounces.

Exchange Values Per Serving:
1 Vegetable
½ Fat

47 Calories
(38% from Fat)
7.6gm Carbohydrates
1.3gm Protein
2gm Fat
0mg Cholesterol
613mg Sodium
608mg Potassium

Spiced Lowfat Buttermilk

MAKES FOUR SERVINGS

16 ounces lowfat buttermilk
½ teaspoon rum flavoring
Dash nutmeg
Dash cinnamon
Cinnamon sticks

Stir together all of the ingredients except the cinnamon sticks and chill covered. Serve in small glass punch cups and place a stick of cinnamon in each cup. One serving equals 4 ounces.

Exchange Values
Per Serving:
½ Milk

50 Calories
(21% from Fat)
5.9gm Carbohydrates
4gm Protein
1.1gm Fat
5mg Cholesterol
129mg Sodium
186mg Potassium

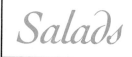

Salads

Eggplant Salad

EIGHT SERVINGS

1 large eggplant
½ cup olive oil
1 cup chopped onion
1 cup chopped celery
1 cup chopped green pepper
1 cup tomato puree
½ cup chopped black olives
½ cup red wine vinegar
2 tablespoons sugar

*Exchange Values
Per Serving:*
2 Vegetable
3 Fat

187 Calories
(70% from Fat)
14.9gm Carbohydrates
1.8gm Protein
14.6gm Fat
0mg Cholesterol
215mg Sodium
394mg Potassium

*C*ut the unpeeled eggplant into small cubes. In a large skillet, heat ½ cup of olive oil over moderately high heat. Sauté the eggplant, turning and stirring until nicely browned, about 10 minutes. Add the onion, celery, and green pepper, and cook all crisp-tender. Stir in the tomato puree, olives, vinegar, and sugar. Simmer uncovered for 10 minutes, stirring occasionally. Remove from the heat. Cool and refrigerate. This is great served with crackers, pita bread triangles, and even tortilla squares.

Celery Cole Slaw

3 cups finely shredded cabbage
3 tablespoons olive oil
⅓ cup warm vinegar
1 tablespoon finely chopped onion
1 tablespoon chopped pimiento
2 packets artificial sweetener
½ teaspoon dry mustard
½ teaspoon celery seeds

Exchange Values
Per Serving:
1 Vegetable
2 Fat

110 Calories
(84% from Fat)
5.8gm Carbohydrates
0.9gm Protein
10.3gm Fat
0mg Cholesterol
13mg Sodium
157mg Potassium

*T*oss the cabbage, oil, and warm vinegar in a bowl. Add the remaining ingredients and toss again. Cover and refrigerate for 2 hours or until time to serve.

Chicken Salad

2 cups cooked brown rice
1½ cups cooked, diced chicken

⅛ teaspoon salt (optional)
½ cup plain lowfat yogurt
2 tablespoons reduced calorie salad dressing
1 garlic clove, minced
1 cup sliced celery
2 teaspoons chopped pimiento
1 cup diced tomatoes
2 tablespoons mustard

Exchange Values
Per Serving:
1 Bread
1½ Meat

153 Calories
(23% from Fat)
14.3gm Carbohydrates
14.6gm Protein
3.9gm Fat
39mg Cholesterol
189mg Sodium
267mg Potassium

*C*ombine the rice and chicken, and chill. Combine the yogurt, salad dressing, and garlic, and mix with the rice and chicken. Add the remaining ingredients and toss lightly. Serve on lettuce or inside chilled, hollowed green peppers (not calculated in analysis).

Tuna Salad

2 7-ounce cans tuna, packed in water, drained
1 cup plain lowfat yogurt
2 Kosher pickle spears, finely diced
½ cup finely cut celery
   Pinch garlic salt
   Pinch paprika
1 tablespoon mustard

   ▪ ▪ ▪

   Crisp lettuce

Exchange Values
Per Serving:
2½ Meat

104 Calories
(11% from Fat)
3.6gm Carbohydrates
19.1gm Protein
1.2gm Fat
41.9mg Cholesterol
499mg Sodium
325mg Potassium

*C*ombine all of the ingredients except the lettuce in a bowl. Mix well. Chill for 2 hours. With an ice cream scoop, scoop out servings and place on a lettuce leaf.

Fresh Broccoli and Cauliflower Salad

1 bunch fresh broccoli
8 ounces fresh mushrooms
1 bunch fresh cauliflower
4 ounces fresh cherry tomatoes

   ▪ ▪ ▪

⅓ cup safflower oil
½ cup red wine vinegar
½ teaspoon parsley flakes
1 teaspoon onion, minced
½ teaspoon minced garlic clove
½ teaspoon poppy seeds
   Dash pepper

Exchange Values
Per Serving:
3 Vegetable
2 Fat

166 Calories
(54% from Fat)
17.3gm Carbohydrates
7.6gm Protein
10.0gm Fat
0mg Cholesterol
59mg Sodium
1116mg Potassium

*M*ix the fresh vegetables in a large bowl. Spoon onto individual plates.

Combine the remaining ingredients for the dressing and pour over the fresh vegetables. Toss gently.

Turkey Salad with Cantaloupe

TWELVE SERVINGS

1¼ cups uncooked rice
2 large cantaloupes
3 tablespoons oil
4 teaspoons orange juice
4 teaspoons vinegar
½ teaspoon grated orange peel
4 cups cubed, cooked turkey or chicken
1 cup diced celery
1 cup red seedless grapes
¾ cup reduced-calorie mayonnaise

   ■ ■ ■

¾ cup cashew halves
12 cantaloupe wedges
   Lettuce leaves

*Exchange Values
Per Serving:*
1 Fruit
1 Bread
2½ Meat
2 Fat

*350 Calories
(41% from Fat)*
33.4gm Carbohydrates
20.7gm Protein
15.2gm Fat
49mg Cholesterol
151mg Sodium
701mg Potassium

Cook the rice according to the package directions. Drain, rinse with cold water, and set aside. Cut each cantaloupe into six wedges and remove the seeds. Remove the rind and cut the melon into 1-inch pieces. Measure 3 cups. Combine the oil, orange juice, vinegar, and orange peel in a large bowl. Blend well. Add the turkey, stirring to coat. Add 3 cups of cantaloupe, the celery, grapes, and mayonnaise, and mix well. Cover and refrigerate until thoroughly chilled. Just before serving, stir in the cashew halves. Place cantaloupe wedges on lettuce-lined serving plates and spoon ¾ cup of salad into each wedge.

Green Bean Salad

FOUR SERVINGS

1 10-ounce package frozen cut green beans
4 teaspoons safflower oil
¼ cup water
¼ cup white wine vinegar with tarragon
1 teaspoon sugar
   Dash pepper
⅛ teaspoon paprika

*Exchange Values
Per Serving:*
1 Vegetable
1 Fat

*74 Calories
(58% from Fat)*

½ teaspoon dry mustard
½ teaspoon Worcestershire sauce
1 clove garlic, minced (optional)
1 tablespoon finely chopped onion
2 teaspoons finely chopped parsley

7.8gm Carbohydrates
1.4gm Protein
4.8gm Fat
0mg Cholesterol
9mg Sodium
153mg Potassium

Cook the green beans according to the package directions. Drain and set aside. Combine the remaining ingredients and blend well. Pour the mixture over the green beans and refrigerate for a few hours or until ready to serve. When ready to serve, drain the green beans and arrange on salad plates.

House Salad with Dream Pepper Dressing

THREE SERVINGS

½ head iceberg lettuce
½ head romaine lettuce

■ ■ ■

2–3 rings sliced jumbo onions
2–3 rings sliced green peppers
2–3 rings sliced cucumbers
3 tomato wedges

■ ■ ■

1 quart reduced calorie mayonnaise
1 cup water
1½ tablespoons Parmesan cheese
2½ teaspoons peppercorn
2½ teaspoons Mrs. Dash herbs
Dash Tabasco
2½ teaspoons vinegar
1 tablespoon diced onion
Dash garlic powder
2½ teaspoons lemon juice
1 teaspoon soy sauce

*Exchange Values
Per Salad
Serving:*
1½ Vegetable

39 Calories
(10% from Fat)
7.2gm Carbohydrates
2.9gm Protein
0.5gm Fat
0mg Cholesterol
17.6mg Sodium
516.6mg Potassium

*Exchange Values
Per Dressing
Tablespoonful:*
1½ Fat

65 Calories
(93% from Fat)
1.1gm Carbohydrates
0.2gm Protein
6.7gm Fat
8mg Cholesterol
137mg Sodium
2mg Potassium

Hand break the lettuces and mix. Chill. When ready to serve place on each of 3 salad plates 1 cup of lettuce, 1 ring of onion, 1 ring of green pepper, 1 ring of cucumber, and a tomato wedge.

Mix the remaining ingredients in a blender on high until thoroughly blended. Ladle over the lettuce by the tablespoon.

Old-Fashioned Potato Salad

SIX SERVINGS

2 cups diced cooked potatoes
½ cup finely chopped onion
¼ cup finely cut celery
1 whole dill pickle, finely chopped

■ ■ ■

½ cup plain lowfat yogurt
1 tablespoon prepared mustard
¾ teaspoon "no oil" herb or Italian seasoning

Exchange Values
Per Serving:
1 Bread

73 Calories
(5% from Fat)
14.8gm Carbohydrates
2.3gm Protein
0.4gm Fat
1.2mg Cholesterol
208mg Sodium
333mg Potassium

Combine the potatoes, onion, celery, and pickle. In a small bowl, combine the yogurt, mustard and seasonings. Add to the vegetables and mix carefully. Cover and refrigerate for several hours to allow the flavors to blend.

Skillet Apple Potato Salad

FOUR SERVINGS

4 medium red potatoes
4 slices bacon, diced
¼ cup chopped green onions
¼ cup chopped green pepper
¼ cup water
½ cup cider vinegar
1 tablespoon sugar
¼ teaspoon paprika
¼ teaspoon dry mustard
3 large Golden Delicious apples, cored and coarsely diced

Exchange Values
Per Serving:
1 Bread
1 Fat
2 Fruits

289 Calories
(19% from Fat)
59gm Carbohydrates
6.5gm Protein
6.0gm Fat
5.0mg Cholesterol
85.8mg Sodium
818mg Potassium

Wash the potatoes and cook in the skins in boiling water just until tender. Drain and coarsely dice. Sauté the bacon in a large heavy skillet until crisp. Add the green onions and green pepper and sauté for a few minutes. Drain. Stir in the water, vinegar, sugar, paprika, and mustard. Heat to boiling. Add the potatoes and apples to the skillet and heat through, stirring gently. Serve immediately.

Spinach Salad

FOUR SERVINGS

1 bunch spinach, washed and stems removed
¼ pound bean sprouts
¼ pound scallops
1 clove garlic, minced
⅛ teaspoon Mrs. Dash seasoned salt substitute
1 tablespoon cider vinegar
⅛ cup sliced fresh mushrooms
⅛ tablespoon pimiento
   Dash pepper

Exchange Values
Per Serving:
½ Vegetable
½ Meat

34 Calories
(10% from Fat)
2.6gm Carbohydrates
5.8gm Protein
0.4gm Fat
10mg Cholesterol
74mg Sodium
335mg Potassium

*T*oss all of the ingredients together in a salad bowl. Cover and chill before serving.

Molded Cucumber Salad

SIX SERVINGS

1 ¼-ounce envelope unflavored gelatin
¼ cup cold water
¼ teaspoon salt substitute
⅛ teaspoon white pepper
¼ teaspoon finely grated dill weed
2 tablespoons grated onion
2 large cucumbers, chilled
1 cup plain lowfat yogurt

Exchange Values
Per Serving:
½ Milk
½ Vegetable

41 Calories
(15% from Fat)
5.6gm Carbohydrates
3.5gm Protein
0.7gm Fat
2.3mg Cholesterol
30mg Sodium
372mg Potassium

*S*often the gelatin in the cold water. Heat the water to boiling to dissolve the gelatin. Allow to cool to lukewarm. Add the salt substitute, pepper, dill weed, and onion. Thinly slice the cucumbers and add to the mix. Stir well. Add the yogurt to the mixture and pour into a mold. Refrigerate for 4 hours. Serve on a lettuce leaf.

Pasta Salad

SIX SERVINGS

1 12-ounce package Rainbow or Garden Style Twirls, uncooked
¾ cup creamy Dijon dressing
1 cup cherry tomato halves
¾ cup ground cooked turkey
   Lettuce

Cook the twirls according to the package directions. Drain and rinse with cold water to cool quickly. In a medium bowl toss the twirls with the dressing. Stir in the tomatoes and turkey just until blended. Serve in lettuce lined bowls. Top with additional dressing, if desired.

Exchange Values
Per Serving:
1 Vegetable
2 Bread
1 Meat
2 Fat

328 Calories
(38% from Fat)
35.8gm Carbohydrates
14.9gm Protein
13.9gm Fat
73.6mg Cholesterol
337mg Sodium
456mg Potassium

Gazpacho Salad

SIX SERVINGS

1¾ cups crushed tomatoes
⅓ cup chopped onion
2 cloves garlic, minced
1 tablespoon chopped fresh parsley
½ teaspoon sugar
½ teaspoon chopped chives
½ teaspoon basil leaves
½ teaspoon red hot sauce

■ ■ ■

1 12-ounce package Rainbow or Garden Style shells, uncooked
1 tablespoon olive oil
2 cups diced cucumber
1 cup thinly sliced green pepper
½ cup sliced celery

Exchange Values
Per Serving:
1 Vegetable
2 Bread
½ Fat

259 Calories
(11% from Fat)
49.2gm Carbohydrates
8.2gm Protein
3.2gm Fat
0mg Cholesterol
23mg Sodium
378mg Potassium

To make the dressing, combine the tomatoes, onion, garlic, parsley, sugar, chives, basil, and red hot sauce in a small bowl. Cover and refrigerate until needed.

Cook the shells according to package directions. Drain and rinse with cold water to cool quickly. In a large bowl, toss the shells with oil. Add the cucumber, pepper, and celery. Toss lightly. Top each portion with dressing before serving.

Macaroni Salad

3 cups hot cooked macaroni, drained
⅓ cup thinly sliced celery
1 tablespoon chopped green onions
1 cup chopped cooked green onions
1 cup chopped cooked broccoli
1 cup chopped cooked cauliflower

■ ■ ■

½ cup plain lowfat yogurt
1 tablespoon prepared mustard
¾ teaspoon "no oil" herb or Italian seasoning

Exchange Values
Per Serving:
1 Vegetable
1 Bread

125 Calories
(6% from Fat)
24.1gm Carbohydrates
5.7gm Protein
0.9gm Fat
1.2mg Cholesterol
60mg Sodium
286mg Potassium

Combine the macaroni and vegetables. Combine the yogurt, mustard and seasoning in a separate bowl and mix well. Add to the vegetable and macaroni mixture and chill.

Tangy Tomato Aspic

2 3-ounce packages sugar-free lemon gelatin
1½ cups boiling water

■ ■ ■

2 cups pure tomato juice
1 bay leaf
1 stalk celery, sliced
1 small onion, sliced
⅛ teaspoon pepper

■ ■ ■

¼ cup finely chopped celery

Exchange Values
Per Serving:
1 Vegetable

32 Calories
(3% from Fat)
5.3gm Carbohydrates
2.1gm Protein
0.1gm Fat
0mg Cholesterol
314mg Sodium
400mg Potassium

Dissolve the gelatin in boiling water. Warm the tomato juice and simmer with the bay leaf, sliced celery, onion, and pepper. Strain the tomato juice mixture and combine with the gelatin. Refrigerate until the mixture begins to thicken. Add the finely chopped celery and stir. Chill until firm. Cut into squares.

Pasta and Vegetable Salad

12 ounces medium shell macaroni
1 small zucchini cut into 1-inch julienne strips
½ cup shredded carrots
1 cup steamed broccoli
¼ cup pimientos
2 tablespoons chopped Italian parsley

   ■ ■ ■

¼ cup plain lowfat yogurt
2 tablespoons red wine vinegar
1 tablespoon liquid oil
1 garlic clove, minced
½ teaspoon crushed oregano
¼ teaspoon crushed basil
¼ teaspoon salt substitute
⅛ teaspoon pepper

Exchange Values
Per Serving:
1 Vegetable
3 Bread
1 Fat

376 Calories
(11% from Fat)
70.0gm Carbohydrates
12.7gm Protein
4.5gm Fat
0.9mg Cholesterol
22mg Sodium
409mg Potassium

*P*repare the macaroni according to the package directions, without salt. Combine the cooked macaroni, zucchini, carrot, broccoli, pimientos, and Italian parsley. Combine the remaining ingredients, and pour over the salad. Cover and chill about 1 hour.

Wild Rice Salad

1 6-ounce package wild rice mix

   ■ ■ ■

½ cup reduced calorie mayonnaise
⅓ cup plain lowfat yogurt
1 cup celery, sliced
1 cup tomato, cubed
½ cup cucumber, diced

Exchange Values
Per Serving:
1 Bread
1 Fat

113 Calories
(47% from Fat)

2 tablespoons parsley, chopped
⅛ teaspoon Mrs. Dash seasoned salt substitute
⅛ teaspoon pepper

13.3gm Carbohydrates
2gm Protein
6gm Fat
7.4mg Cholesterol
30mg Sodium
207mg Potassium

Cook the rice according to the package directions, omitting margarine. Cool. Toss lightly with the remaining ingredients. Cover and chill.

Red Pepper and Pasta Salad

FOUR SERVINGS

1 medium red bell pepper, seeded and cut into fourths

■ ■ ■

2 cups uncooked rotini

■ ■ ■

2 cups fresh spinach, cut into thin strips
1 cup sliced zucchini
½ cup thinly sliced carrot
½ cup bottled low-calorie Italian dressing
2 tablespoons chopped fresh parsley
2 tablespoons lemon juice
1 teaspoon grated lemon peel
1 cup plain lowfat yogurt

Exchange Values
Per Serving:
2 Vegetable
2 Bread
½ Fat

253 Calories
(6% from Fat)
49.0gm Carbohydrates
10.4gm Protein
1.8gm Fat
1mg Cholesterol
584mg Sodium
581mg Potassium

Place the red pepper quarters on a broiler pan, skin side up. Broil 3 to 4 inches from the heat until the skin blackens, then remove from the broiler. Place in a plastic bag, and let stand for 10 minutes to steam. Peel the skin from the pepper, and cut each piece into ½-inch pieces. Cook the rotini according to the package directions. Drain, and rinse with cold water. Combine all of the ingredients in a large bowl. Cover and refrigerate for several hours or overnight.

Apple Nut Salad

FOUR SERVINGS

½ cup cold water
1 .3-ounce package sugar-free apple gelatin
2 tablespoons freshly squeezed lemon juice
1 cup apple juice or clear cider

■ ■ ■

1 medium apple
¼ cup chopped pecans

■ ■ ■

Nondairy whipped topping

Exchange Values
Per Serving:
1½ Fruits
1 Fat

133 Calories
(51% from Fat)
15.6gm Carbohydrates
2.3gm Protein
7.6gm Fat
0mg Cholesterol
11mg Sodium
204mg Potassium

*B*ring the water to a boil in a small saucepan. Add the gelatin and stir until dissolved. Stir in the lemon and apple juices.

Remove from the heat and chill until the mixture is as thick as unbeaten egg whites. Core and cube the unpeeled apple, and add it to the gelatin. Add the nuts and fold together. Turn the mixture into a 3-cup mold that has been rinsed in cold water and chill until set. Unmold onto a platter, garnish, and serve with 2 tablespoons nondairy whipped topping on each serving.

Apple-Orange Cider Salad

EIGHT SERVINGS

1 6-ounce package sugar-free orange gelatin
4 cups apple cider

■ ■ ■

1 cup raisins
1 cup coarsely chopped apple
1 cup chopped celery
Juice and grated rind of 1 lemon

Exchange Values
Per Serving:
2 Fruit

134 Calories
(1% from Fat)
32.8gm Carbohydrates
2.3gm Protein
0.2gm Fat
0mg Cholesterol
27mg Sodium
398mg Potassium

*D*issolve the gelatin in 2 cups of hot cider. Stir in the raisins and allow the mixture to cool. Add the remaining cider. Chill until slightly thickened. Add the remaining ingredients and chill until set.

Christmas Salad

1 3-ounce package sugar-free lemon gelatin
2 cups boiling water
1 6-ounce can unsweetened orange juice concentrate
1 cup ground raw cranberries (measure after grinding)
2 teaspoons grated orange rind
1 8-ounce can unsweetened crushed pineapple
1 cup broken pecans

Exchange Values Per Serving:
2 Fat
1 Fruit

155 Calories
(54% from Fat)
17.4gm Carbohydrates
2.5gm Protein
9.2gm Fat
0mg Cholesterol
13mg Sodium
241mg Potassium

*D*issolve the gelatin in the boiling water. Add the orange juice concentrate and stir. Add the remaining ingredients, including the cranberries. Pour into a mold. This is best when prepared a day in advance.

Fluffy Orange Yogurt Salad

1 20-ounce can pineapple chunks, drained
1 16-ounce can mandarin orange segments, drained
1 cup nondairy whipped topping
4 ounces or ½ cup orange- or pineapple-flavored lowfat yogurt

2 bananas, sliced

Exchange Values Per Serving:
2 Fruit

118 Calories
(21% from Fat)
22.8gm Carbohydrates
1.5gm Protein
2.8gm Fat
0.9mg Cholesterol
19mg Sodium
309mg Potassium

*I*n a medium bowl, combine pineapple and orange segments. Combine the whipped topping and yogurt in a blender until fluffy. Gently toss the topping with the pineapple and orange fruits. Cover and place in the refrigerator for 2 hours or more. Just before serving gently add the bananas. Spoon into tall wine glasses and top with a mint leaf.

Fruit and Nut Curried Salad

EIGHT SERVINGS

1 head red leaf or romaine lettuce, torn
1 cup torn fresh spinach
1 cup grapes, halved and seeded
1 cup bean sprouts
1 11-ounce can mandarin orange sections, chilled and drained

■ ■ ■

½ cup safflower oil
⅓ cup white wine vinegar
1 clove garlic, minced
2 tablespoons brown sugar substitute
2 tablespoons minced chives
1 tablespoon curry powder
1 teaspoon soy sauce
¼ cup toasted slivered almonds

Exchange Values
Per Serving:
2 Fat
½ Fruit

126 Calories
(67% from Fat)
10.4gm Carbohydrates
2.2gm Protein
9.4gm Fat
0mg Cholesterol
28mg Sodium
235mg Potassium

Combine the red leaf or romaine lettuce, torn spinach, seeded grapes, bean sprouts, and mandarin oranges. Set aside. Combine the oil, vinegar, garlic, brown sugar, chives, curry powder, and soy sauce in a jar. Pour some dressing over salad, tossing lightly to coat. Scatter the almonds over the salad. Serve the remaining dressing with the salad or save for use later. Extra tablespoons are 1 fat exchange each.

Fruit Combo with an Orange Twist

SIXTEEN SERVINGS

3 cups cantaloupe balls or cubes
3 cups fresh pineapple chunks
2 cups halved fresh strawberries

■ ■ ■

¼ cup sugar-free orange marmalade
2 tablespoons lemon juice
2 tablespoons orange-flavored liqueur

Exchange Values
Per Serving:
½ Fruit

43 Calories
(5% from Fat)
9.1gm Carbohydrates
0.5gm Protein
0.3gm Fat
0mg Cholesterol
3mg Sodium
161mg Potassium

Combine the fruits in a large bowl and toss gently. Combine the marmalade, lemon juice, and orange liqueur, and mix well. Pour over the fruit mixture, stirring to coat completely. Cover and refrigerate for several hours or overnight, stirring once.

Gingered Fruit Compote

FOUR SERVINGS

1 apple, cored and sectioned
1 orange, sectioned
1 banana, sliced
1 cup green grapes, seedless
¼ cup orange juice
2 teaspoons freshly grated ginger

*C*ombine and mix the fruits and orange juice in a serving dish. Add the ginger and stir well. Refrigerate for at least 2 hours. Serve garnished with mint leaf or with 2 tablespoons nondairy whipped topping.

Exchange Values
Per Serving:
1½ Fruit

88 Calories
(4% from Fat)
22.4gm Carbohydrates
1gm Protein
0.4gm Fat
0mg Cholesterol
2mg Sodium
302mg Potassium

Gingered Pineapple Mold

TEN SERVINGS

1 20-ounce can unsweetened pineapple chunks
1 .6-ounce package sugar-free lime gelatin
1½ cups boiling water
1 cup sugar-free ginger ale
¼ teaspoon ginger

*D*rain the pineapple chunks. Dissolve the gelatin in the boiling water and allow to cool. Add the pineapple chunks, ginger ale, and ginger, and mix well. Pour into a mold and refrigerate for 4 hours or until completely set.

Exchange Values
Per Serving:
½ Fruit

24 Calories
(4% from Fat)
4.8gm Carbohydrates
1.4gm Protein
0.1gm Fat
0mg Cholesterol
11mg Sodium
106mg Potassium

Mellow Ambrosia

FOUR SERVINGS

2 medium oranges, peeled and diced
1 small banana, sliced
¼ cup orange juice
2 tablespoons wheat germ

Combine the fruits and juice, and portion into dessert dishes. Sprinkle with wheat germ.

*Exchange Values
Per Serving:*
1 Fruit

66 Calories
(8% from Fat)
15.3gm Carbohydrates
2.0gm Protein
0.6gm Fat
0mg Cholesterol
0.5mg Sodium
284mg Potassium

Molded Tart Apple Salad

FOUR SERVINGS

1 .3-ounce package sugar-free strawberry gelatin
¾ cup boiling water
½ cup apple cider
Ice cubes
1 medium apple, sliced and wedged

Dissolve the gelatin in the boiling water. Combine the cider and ice cubes to make 1¼ cups. Add to the gelatin and stir until slightly thickened, then remove any unmelted ice. Pour into a mold. Place the apple wedges in the gelatin. Chill for about 2 hours to set.

*Exchange Values
Per Serving:*
½ Fruit

42 Calories
(4% from Fat)
8.9gm Carbohydrates
1.5gm Protein
0.2gm Fat
0mg Cholesterol
9mg Sodium
118mg Potassium

Orange Pineapple Salad

1   16-ounce can mandarin oranges
1   16-ounce can unsweetened crushed pineapple
1   6-ounce package sugar-free orange gelatin
1   8-ounce carton nondairy whipped topping
1   8-ounce carton lowfat cottage cheese

*D*rain the juices from the oranges and pineapple into a saucepan. Heat to the boiling point, and remove from the heat. Mix in the gelatin, stirring until dissolved. When the gelatin has cooled, stir in the fruits, whipped topping, and cottage cheese. Refrigerate overnight before serving.

Exchange Values Per Serving:
1 Fruit
1 Meat

117 Calories
(23% from Fat)
17.6gm Carbohydrates
6.0gm Protein
3.0gm Fat
2mg Cholesterol
129mg Sodium
215mg Potassium

Peaches and Cream Salad

1   3-ounce package sugar-free peach gelatin
1   cup boiling water
⅓   cup sugar-free ginger ale
½   cup plain lowfat yogurt
1¾ cups thawed nondairy whipped topping
¼   cup chopped walnuts
1   16-ounce can unsweetened sliced peaches, drained and chopped

*D*issolve the gelatin in boiling water. Add cold ginger ale. Chill until slightly thickened. Blend the yogurt into the whipped topping and then fold into the peach gelatin. Stir in the walnuts and peaches, and pour into a loaf pan. Chill until firm, approximately 4 hours. Unmold and garnish with peach slices.

Exchange Values Per Serving:
½ Fruit
1 Fat

102 Calories
(59% from Fat)
9.0gm Carbohydrates
2.4gm Protein
6.7gm Fat
0.1mg Cholesterol
22mg Sodium
132mg Potassium

Pudding Salad

SIX SERVINGS

1 cup lowfat buttermilk
1 8-ounce carton nondairy whipped topping, thawed
1 1.3-ounce package sugar-free vanilla instant pudding mix
1 16-ounce can mandarin oranges, drained
1 16-ounce can unsweetened crushed pineapple

Combine the buttermilk, whipped topping, and pudding mix. Stir in the oranges and pineapple. Cover and refrigerate until ready to serve.

Exchange Values Per Serving:
1½ Fruit
1 Milk

141 Calories
(23% from Fat)
29.5gm Carbohydrates
2.3gm Protein
3.6gm Fat
1.5mg Cholesterol
97mg Sodium
257mg Potassium

Strawberry Gelatin Salad

EIGHT SERVINGS

2 .3-ounce packages sugar-free strawberry gelatin
2 cups boiling water
1 13½-ounce can unsweetened crushed pineapple, undrained
2 10-ounce packages frozen strawberries
1 cup chopped pecans (optional, not in analysis)
2 tablespoons lemon juice

• • •

1 8-ounce container nondairy whipped topping

Dissolve the gelatin in the boiling water. Add the crushed pineapple, juice and all. Add the strawberries, pecans, and lemon juice. Pour into a 2-quart dish and refrigerate overnight. When set, combine the gelatin with half of the whipped topping in a blender, and whip until well blended. Spoon into tall wine glasses, top with the remaining topping and a fresh strawberry.

Exchange Values Per Serving:
1 Fruit

91 Calories
(25% from Fat)
16.4gm Carbohydrates
2.0gm Protein
2.5gm Fat
0mg Cholesterol
13mg Sodium
210mg Potassium

Tropical Fruit Salad

2   kiwi fruit, pared, halved lengthwise, and sliced
1½ cups strawberries, quartered
1   fresh pineapple, cored and sliced in ¼-inch pieces (3 cups)
2   bananas, sliced
1   cup seedless grapes
4   apples, peeled, cored, and cubed
1   cup honeydew melon balls
1   cup cantaloupe melon balls
½   cup pineapple juice
6   medium papayas, halved lengthwise and seeded

■ ■ ■

2   cups nondairy whipped topping
8   ounces pineapple lowfat, low-calorie yogurt

Exchange Values
Per Serving:
3 Fruit

184 Calories
(17% from Fat)
39.0gm Carbohydrates
2.8gm Protein
3.5gm Fat
1.0mg Cholesterol
23mg Sodium
686mg Potassium

Combine the fruits in a bowl and add the juice. Strain and spoon into the papaya halves. Whip together the whipped topping and pineapple yogurt. Place a dollop of whipped mixture over each filled papaya and serve.

Very Orange Salad

½   cup white currants
2   tablespoons unsweetened orange juice

■ ■ ■

4   cups finely shredded carrots
1   cup drained mandarin orange slices
¼   cup drained crushed pineapple
½   cup vanilla lowfat yogurt

Exchange Values
Per Serving:
1 Vegetable
1½ Fruit

103 Calories
(4% from Fat)
24.3gm Carbohydrates
2.5gm Protein
0.5gm Fat
1.2mg Cholesterol
42mg Sodium
463mg Potassium

Place the currants in a bowl. Pour the juice over the currants, and set aside for 5 minutes. Then add the carrots, orange slices and pineapple. Add yogurt and mix well.

Zesty Cranberry Salad

FOUR SERVINGS

2   3-ounce packages sugar-free strawberry gelatin
2½ cups boiling water
1   cup sugar-free lemon lime soda
1   orange
½   cup chopped celery
¼   cup chopped walnuts
1   cup ground cranberries
1   cup crushed unsweetened pineapple

Exchange Values
Per Serving:
1 Fruit
1 Fat

118 Calories
(37% from Fat)
15.6gm Carbohydrates
4.8gm Protein
4.8gm Fat
0mg Cholesterol
40mg Sodium
326mg Potassium

Dissolve the gelatin in boiling water and cool. Grind the entire orange in a food processor. Add the celery, walnuts, and cranberries, and pulsate until chunky. Pour into the gelatin mix and stir. Add the crushed pineapple and lemon lime soda. Stir and refrigerate. This is best when prepared a day in advance.

Buttermilk-Style Dressing

TWENTY-FOUR TABLESPOONFULS

½ cup plain lowfat yogurt
1 cup lowfat cottage cheese
¼ cup finely chopped onion
2 tablespoons finely chopped parsley
1 garlic clove, finely chopped
½ teaspoon paprika

Exchange Values
Per Tablespoon:
Free

13 Calories
(34% from Fat)
0.7gm Carbohydrates
1.5gm Protein
0.5gm Fat
1.7mg Cholesterol
42mg Sodium
24mg Potassium

Whip the yogurt and cottage cheese together until smooth and the consistency of mayonnaise. Add the remaining ingredients and stir well. Refrigerate. This dressing improves with time, and is best made the day before it is to be used. Use up to 2 tablespoons several times a day.

Cottage Cheese Ranch Dressing

TWENTY TABLESPOONFULS

1   cup lowfat cottage cheese
¼ cup skim milk
2   teaspoons Worcestershire sauce
1   tablespoon powdered Hidden Valley Ranch Dressing

*P*lace all of the ingredients in a blender and blend for 2 to 3 minutes or until the mixture has a smooth consistency and is thoroughly blended. Place in a covered storage container and chill until ready to use. Use up to 2 tablespoons several times a day.

Exchange Values Per Tablespoon:
Free

12 Calories
(18% from Fat)
0.7gm Carbohydrates
1.7gm Protein
0.2gm Fat
1mg Cholesterol
106mg Sodium
26mg Potassium

Herbed Spice Dressing

FOUR TABLESPOONFULS

2   tablespoons plain lowfat yogurt
2   tablespoons reduced-calorie mayonnaise
½ teaspoon powdered garlic
½ teaspoon parsley
1   teaspoon Parmesan cheese
½ teaspoon Italian seasoning
    Pinch pepper

*B*lend all of the ingredients together. This is best if refrigerated overnight before using.

Exchange Values Per Tablespoon:
½ Fat

31 Calories
(73% from Fat)
1.3gm Carbohydrates
0.7gm Protein
2.5gm Fat
4mg Cholesterol
59mg Sodium
28mg Potassium

Tartar Sauce Dressing

THIRTY-TWO TABLESPOONFULS

¾ cup chili sauce
1 cup plain lowfat yogurt
1 tablespoon grated onion
¼ cup minced kosher dill pickle spears
1 teaspoon lemon juice
1 teaspoon Worcestershire sauce
½ teaspoon soy sauce
½ teaspoon horseradish

Exchange Values
Per Tablespoon:
Free

11 Calories
(9% from Fat)
2gm Carbohydrates
0.5gm Protein
0.1gm Fat
0.4mg Cholesterol
105mg Sodium
43mg Potassium

Combine all of the ingredients and blend well. Serve with seafood or a seafood salad. Use up to 2 tablespoons several times a day.

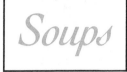

Soups

Beef and Barley Soup

TEN SERVINGS

2 pounds round steak, cubed
1 tablespoon oil

■ ■ ■

8 cups water
3 bouillon cubes
1 28-ounce can whole tomatoes
1 large onion
1 clove garlic

■ ■ ■

1 cup chopped carrots
1 cup chopped celery
⅔ cup barley
  Parsley
⅛ teaspoon pepper
1 teaspoon basil
½ teaspoon Worcestershire sauce
½ teaspoon soy sauce

*Exchange Values
Per Serving:*
1 Vegetable
2 Meat
1 Fat

221 Calories
(29% from Fat)
17.0gm Carbohydrates
21.9gm Protein
7.2gm Fat
56mg Cholesterol
205mg Sodium
609mg Potassium

*I*n a skillet, brown the round steak in oil. Stir in the water, bouillon cubes, undrained tomatoes, onion, and garlic. Simmer for 2 hours. Add the carrots, celery, barley, and seasonings. Continue to simmer for 30 more minutes or until the vegetables are tender.

Chicken and Vegetable Soup

TEN SERVINGS

Uncooked chicken giblets
4½ cups water

■ ■ ■

⅛ teaspoon pepper
2 carrots
1 small onion
2 stalks celery, chopped
1 cup fresh mushrooms
1 6-ounce can tomato juice
1 tablespoon chopped parsley
¼ teaspoon paprika
2 cups cooked, diced chicken breast meat

Exchange Values Per Serving:
1 Meat
1 Vegetable

90 Calories
(19% from Fat)
3.8gm Carbohydrates
14.7gm Protein
1.7gm Fat
39mg Cholesterol
108mg Sodium
290mg Potassium

*W*ash the giblets and discard all fat. Place in a large cooking pot with water. Bring to a boil and simmer for about 25 minutes. Strain out and discard the giblets. Add the remaining ingredients except the chicken. Simmer gently for about 30 minutes or until the vegetables are tender. Add the chicken pieces and stir. Simmer about 10 minutes.

Beef Stew Base

EIGHT SERVINGS

2 pounds stew beef
2 medium onions, sliced
1 chopped green pepper
¾ cup pureed whole tomatoes
¾ cup water
1½ teaspoons Mrs. Dash
⅛ teaspoon pepper
1 tablespoon Worcestershire sauce

Exchange Values Per Serving:
½ Vegetable
3 Meat

197 Calories
(26% from Fat)
5.9gm Carbohydrates
29.6gm Protein
5.6gm Fat
66mg Cholesterol
167mg Sodium
379mg Potassium

*P*lace the stewing beef, onion, and green pepper in a baking dish. Puree the tomatoes in a food processor. Stir in the tomatoes, the water, salt substitute, pepper, Worcestershire sauce and any vegetables desired for a baked beef stew. Bake at 350° for 1 hour or until the vegetables are tender. This can be served over rice.

Family Beef Stew

EIGHT SERVINGS

1¼ pounds top round steak, cubed
1   tablespoon oil

• • •

¼   cup all-purpose flour
⅛   teaspoon black pepper
1   clove garlic
3   cups water with 1 bouillon cube, dissolved
1   teaspoon Worcestershire sauce
1   teaspoon soy sauce
2   cups pared, cubed potatoes
1   cup diced onions
1   cup diced carrots
1   teaspoon Italian seasoning

Exchange Values Per Serving:
½ Vegetable
1 Bread
2 Meat
1 Fat

244 Calories
(53% from Fat)
12.9gm Carbohydrates
15.4gm Protein
14.3gm Fat
49mg Cholesterol
213mg Sodium
578mg Potassium

*B*rown the outside of the round steak cubes in oil. Drain on a paper towel. Combine the remaining ingredients in a large pot and bring to a boil. Lower the temperature to a simmer and cook for 1 hour. Add the meat and pan drippings to the pot and simmer for 30 more minutes. The stew is done when the vegetables are tender.

Oyster Stew

SIX SERVINGS

1   pint oysters and oyster liquid
1   large Vidalia onion, chopped
1   stalk celery
1   small clove garlic, minced
1   tablespoon liquid margarine
2   cups skim milk
⅛   teaspoon cayenne pepper
    Chopped fresh parsley leaves

Exchange Values Per Serving:
½ Milk
1 Meat

85 Calories
(32% from Fat)
8.4gm Carbohydrates
5.8gm Protein
3.0gm Fat
21mg Cholesterol
173mg Sodium
275mg Potassium

*S*auté the onion, celery, and garlic in the butter. Add the oysters and liquid to the sautéed vegetables. Add the milk and pepper. Simmer, but do not boil. Garnish with the parsley.

Gingered Parsnip and Chicken Soup

EIGHT SERVINGS

2 medium white onions
2 tablespoons liquid margarine
8 medium parsnips, peeled and sliced
2 tablespoons grated fresh ginger (or 1 tablespoon powdered)
   Pepper to taste
4 cups chicken broth
1 cup cooked white chicken breast meat
   Chopped parsley

*P*eel and roughly chop the onions. Sauté the onions in a heavy pan with margarine until translucent. Add the parsnips to the onion and sauté. Add the ginger and pepper. Stir for about 1 minute. Add the chicken stock and the meat. Simmer until the parsnips become soft. Drain the mixture, reserving the liquid, and puree parsnips in a food processor. Return the puree to the liquid and simmer for 10 minutes. Adjust the seasonings and serve. Garnish with chopped parsley.

*Exchange Values
Per Serving:*
½ Vegetable
1 Bread
1 Meat
1 Fat

212 Calories
(23% from Fat)
28.2gm Carbohydrates
13.4gm Protein
5.4gm Fat
24mg Cholesterol
453mg Sodium
763mg Potassium

Spicy Crab Soup

SIX SERVINGS

2 cups water
1 10¾-ounce can low-sodium chicken broth
2 16-ounce cans tomatoes, chopped and undrained
¾ cup celery, chopped
¾ cup onion, diced
1 teaspoon seafood seasoning
¼ teaspoon lemon-pepper
1 10-ounce package frozen broccoli, thawed
1 10-ounce package frozen green beans, thawed
1 pound crabmeat, cooked, flaked, and cartilage removed

*Exchange Values
Per Serving:*
2½ Vegetable
2 Meat

147 Calories
(13% from Fat)
15.1gm Carbohydrates
18.5gm Protein
2.3gm Fat

*I*n a 6-quart soup pot, combine the water, broth, tomatoes, celery, onion, seafood seasoning, and lemon-pepper. Bring to a boil and simmer for 20 to 30 minutes. Add the broccoli and beans and simmer for 10 minutes. Add the crabmeat and heat through. Serve immediately.

75.6mg Cholesterol
660mg Sodium
662mg Potassium

Hot Hot Gumbo

EIGHT SERVINGS

⅓ cup all-purpose flour for dredging
  Pepper and paprika to taste
4 chicken breasts, skinned and boned (5 ounces each)
3 tablespoons safflower oil
  ▪ ▪ ▪
1 cup chopped onion
1 cup chopped green pepper
1 28-ounce can tomatoes, skinned
2 pounds sliced okra
8 drops Tabasco sauce
  ▪ ▪ ▪
3 cups cooked wild rice
  Chopped green onion and/or chopped fresh parsley

Exchange Values
Per Serving:
1 Vegetable
1 Bread
2 Meat
1 Fat

283 Calories
(24% from Fat)
31.3gm Carbohydrates
22.9gm Protein
7.7gm Fat
43mg Cholesterol
230mg Sodium
847mg Potassium

*S*eason the flour with pepper and paprika. Dredge the chicken in the flour mixture and brown in hot oil in a large skillet, turning to brown all sides. Remove and place in a baking dish. Bake at 350° for 20 minutes. Sauté the onion and green pepper in the oil used for the chicken. Stir until limp but not brown. Add the tomatoes, okra, and Tabasco, and cook until tender. Place the chicken on a bed of rice and cover with the tomato and okra mix. Garnish with chopped onion and parsley.

Cajun Shrimp and Oyster Soup

SIX SERVINGS

2 quarts water
2 slices lemon
2 dried red hot chilies
1 bay leaf
½ teaspoon dried thyme
Shrimp shells (reserved from shrimp)
Oyster liquid (reserved from oysters)

■ ■ ■

3 tablespoons oil
¼ cup all-purpose flour
½ cup chopped onion
1 teaspoon minced garlic
¾ cup chopped green pepper
¼ cup chopped parsley
½ teaspoon dried thyme
¼ teaspoon cayenne pepper
¼ teaspoon hot pepper sauce
1 16-ounce can tomatoes, undrained
1 10-ounce package frozen okra, thawed, each cut crosswise into
   5 pieces
1 pound medium shrimp, peeled and deveined (shells used for
   stock)
1 pint shucked oysters, drained (liquid used for stock)
2½ cups hot cooked brown rice

Exchange Values
Per Serving:
1 Vegetable
1 Bread
2 Meat
1 Fat

309 Calories
(30% from Fat)
34.4gm Carbohydrates
19.9gm Protein
10.5gm Fat
147mg Cholesterol
327mg Sodium
678mg Potassium

*T*o make the stock, combine the water, lemon slices, chilies, bay leaf, thyme, shrimp shells, and oyster liquid in large stock pot. Bring to a boil and cook at low, uncovered, until the mixture is reduced to about 3 cups, about 25 to 30 minutes. Strain and discard the seasonings.

Combine the oil and flour in a large heavy pan or Dutch oven. Cook and stir over medium heat until the roux turns a dark, rich, red-brown color but is not scorched, 15 to 20 minutes. Stir in the onion and garlic, and cook until soft, stirring constantly. Add the green pepper, parsley, thyme, cayenne, and hot pepper sauce. Cook and stir 5 minutes longer. Gradually whisk in about 2 cups of warm stock and the tomatoes. Return to a boil and simmer for 20 minutes, stirring occasionally. Add the okra and simmer just until the okra is tender, about 5 minutes. Add the shrimp and oysters. Simmer until the edges of the oysters curl and the shrimp is pink and opaque, 5 to 8 minutes. Do not overcook the seafood. Remove from the heat. Mound the hot rice in soup dishes and ladle the gumbo over the top.

Lentil Bean and Beef Soup

SIXTEEN SERVINGS

2 pounds lean pot roast
⅓ cup soy sauce
■ ■ ■
2 carrots, diced
4 stalks celery, diced
2 large Vidalia onions
1 clove garlic, finely minced
½ cup liquid margarine
■ ■ ■
2 pounds lentils
4 quarts water
Pepper to taste
2 tablespoons parsley leaves, chopped
■ ■ ■
1 28-ounce can whole tomatoes

Exchange Values
Per Serving:
½ Vegetable
2 Meat
2 Fat
2 Bread

356 Calories
(23% from Fat)
38.0gm Carbohydrates
30.6gm Protein
9.1gm Fat
36mg Cholesterol
284mg Sodium
923mg Potassium

Chop the pot roast into 1-inch cubes. Place in a bowl and marinate in soy sauce overnight in the refrigerator.

Sauté the carrots, celery, onion, garlic, and meat in the margarine in a soup kettle. Add the lentils, water, and seasonings, and simmer for 1½ to 2 hours. Puree the whole tomatoes in a food processor and add to the soup mixture. Serve hot.

Meatball Soup

TEN SERVINGS

1 pound lean ground chuck
¼ cup cheese cracker crumbs
1 tablespoon parsley
1 teaspoon minced onion
1 teaspoon oregano
1 teaspoon pepper

■ ■ ■

1 quart unsalted chicken broth
1 pound fresh cut or frozen spinach
1 cup tortellini (available with no cholesterol)

*C*ombine the meat, cracker crumbs, parsley, and seasonings. Shape into small meatballs and brown in the oven. Drain the meatballs and add to the chicken broth along with the spinach. Simmer for 10 minutes. Cook and drain the tortellini. Add to the soup just before serving.

*Exchange Values
Per Serving:*
1 Vegetable
½ Bread
2 Meat
½ Fat

211 Calories
(52% from Fat)
9.9gm Carbohydrates
15.3gm Protein
12.3gm Fat
45.9mg Cholesterol
184mg Sodium
422mg Potassium

Cold Weather Soup

SIX SERVINGS

6 cups water
6 chicken bouillon cubes
2 medium carrots, pared and diced
1 large potato, pared and diced
1 cup cabbage, shredded
2 medium ribs celery, chopped
1 medium onion, chopped
1 small white turnip, chopped
⅛ teaspoon nutmeg
⅛ teaspoon pepper
¼ cup dry white wine

*B*ring the water and bouillon cubes to a boil in a 3 quart stockpot. Add the carrot, potato, cabbage, celery, onion, turnip, nutmeg, and pepper. Bring to a boil, lower the temperature to simmer and add the wine. Simmer until the vegetables are tender, about 25 minutes.

*Exchange Values
Per Serving:*
1 Vegetable
½ Bread

66 Calories
(3% from Fat)
13.1gm Carbohydrates
1.7gm Protein
0.2gm Fat
0mg Cholesterol
814mg Sodium
540mg Potassium

French Onion Soup "In A Hurry"

6   beef bouillon cubes
5   cups boiling water
½   cup pure tomato juice
2   cups fresh onion rings
6   small unsalted melba toast rounds
12 tablespoons grated Parmesan cheese

*D*issolve bouillon cubes in boiling water. Add the tomato juice and onions. Cover and simmer gently for 25 to 30 minutes. Serve in warmed bowls with a melba toast round. Sprinkle 2 tablespoons of Parmesan cheese on top of each.

Exchange Values
Per Serving:
1 Meat
½ Bread

85 Calories
(36% from Fat)
8.3gm Carbohydrates
5.5gm Protein
3.4gm Fat
8mg Cholesterol
1061mg Sodium
172mg Potassium

Carrot and Ginger Soup

1   pound peeled, sliced carrots
1   16-ounce can tomatoes
2   large onions, chopped
1   clove garlic, chopped
½   cup orange juice, unsweetened
2   tablespoons chopped parsley
2   teaspoons seasoned salt substitute
    Pepper to taste
1   teaspoon ginger

½   cup skim milk
¼   cup liquid margarine

*P*lace the carrots, tomatoes, onions, garlic, orange juice, parsley, seasoned salt, pepper and ginger in a large stock pot. Cover with water and cook until tender. Remove from the pot when tender and puree in a food processor. Return to the pot and add the skim milk and margarine. Stir and simmer for approximately 10 more minutes. This can be served in a cleaned out pumpkin and heated in a warm oven for about 5 minutes.

Exchange Values
Per Serving:
1 Vegetable
1 Fat

74 Calories
(58% from Fat)
7.0gm Carbohydrates
1.5gm Protein
4.8gm Fat
0mg Cholesterol
197mg Sodium
236mg Potassium

Vegetable and Pasta Soup

1 cup chopped onion
¾ cup sliced carrots
¾ cup sliced celery
1 clove garlic, minced
3 tablespoons olive oil
6 cups water
1 28-ounce can whole tomatoes in water
1 6-ounce can tomato paste
2 teaspoons Mrs. Dash
3 cups chopped green cabbage
1 cup green beans

■ ■ ■

2 cups cooked tubular vegetable pasta

Exchange Values
Per Serving:
2 Vegetable
1 Bread
1 Fat

165 Calories
(32% from Fat)
24.9gm Carbohydrates
4.8gm Protein
6.2gm Fat
12.5mg Cholesterol
216mg Sodium
679mg Potassium

*P*lace all of the ingredients except the pasta in a large stew pot. Bring to a boil and then reduce the heat to a simmer. Simmer for 1 to 1½ hours or until vegetables are tender. Add the pasta to the soup.

Vegetable Soup

3½ cups boiling water
4   cups whole, skinless tomatoes
2   chicken bouillon cubes
2   beef bouillon cubes
1   large onion, chopped
2   medium carrots, chopped
2   stalks celery, chopped
2   potatoes, skinned and diced
1   clove garlic, minced
1   teaspoon pepper
1   whole turnip
1   cup green beans, canned
1   cup cauliflower, frozen
½   teaspoon crushed sage
1   tablespoon soy sauce

Exchange Values
Per Serving:
2 Vegetable
½ Bread

103 Calories
(8% from Fat)
22.8gm Carbohydrates
4gm Protein
0.75gm Fat
0mg Cholesterol
618mg Sodium
512mg Potassium

Combine all of the ingredients in a large pot. Bring to a boil, stirring to dissolve the bouillon. Cover and simmer gently for 1½ hours. Stir occasionally.

Cream of Chicken and Wild Rice Soup

EIGHT SERVINGS

½   cup wild rice
1   tablespoon soy sauce
1½ cups water

   ■ ■ ■

3   large cloves garlic, minced
1   medium onion, chopped
8   teaspoons margarine
2   carrots, finely diced
6   stalks asparagus, finely diced

   ■ ■ ■

½   cup all-purpose flour

   ■ ■ ■

5   cups chicken stock
½   teaspoon thyme
1   bay leaf
     Minced parsley
     Pepper to taste
1   cup chopped cooked chicken breast
4   cups skim milk

Exchange Values
Per Serving:
½ Milk
½ Vegetable
1 Bread
1 Meat
1 Fat

252 Calories
(24% from Fat)
23.8gm Carbohydrates
19.1gm Protein
6.3gm Fat
27mg Cholesterol
716mg Sodium
567mg Potassium

Cook the wild rice with the soy sauce and water in a covered pan. Sauté the garlic and onion in margarine in a large saucepan until tender. Add the carrots and asparagus and cook until tender. Mix in the flour and cook over low heat for approximately 10 minutes, stirring frequently. Pour in the chicken stock, using a wire whisk to blend until smooth. Add the seasonings and chicken. Slowly add the skim milk. Simmer for 20 minutes. Fold in the prepared rice and serve.

Cream of Broccoli Soup

SIX SERVINGS

2   tablespoons liquid margarine
2   tablespoons all-purpose flour
½   teaspoon salt substitute
    Pepper to taste
1½ cups chicken broth
2   cups lowfat milk
¼   cup nonfat dry milk
10 broccoli spears, cooked

*M*elt the margarine in a saucepan. Stir in the flour, salt substitute, and pepper until blended. Gradually add the chicken broth, stirring over medium heat until the mixture thickens. Add the milk and stir until smooth. Pour the dry milk and 5 broccoli spears into a blender, blend until smooth, and then add to the cooked mixture. Chop the remaining broccoli and add to the soup. Simmer for 5 minutes and serve.

Exchange Values
Per Serving:
½ Milk
2 Vegetable
1 Fat

153 Calories
(34% from Fat)
17gm Carbohydrates
10.2gm Protein
6.2gm Fat
6.8mg Cholesterol
311mg Sodium
712mg Potassium

Cream of Carrot Soup

FOUR SERVINGS

1   leek, sliced
4   teaspoons margarine
2   to 3 carrots, peeled and sliced
1   medium baking potato, cubed
3   quarts chicken broth
4   cups skim milk
    Pepper to taste

*S*auté the leek in margarine in a soup pot or large saucepan until translucent. Add the carrots, potato and stock, cover and bring to a boil. Simmer until the potato and carrots are tender. Place in a blender, reserving some of the liquid for later, and blend until smooth. Strain. Pour the carrot puree back into the soup pot and add the skim milk. Add pepper to taste.

Exchange Values
Per Serving:
1 Vegetable
1 Bread
2 Fat
1 Milk

331 Calories
(23% from Fat)
36.2gm Carbohydrates
25.6gm Protein
8.6gm Fat
5mg Cholesterol
2519mg Sodium
1573mg Potassium

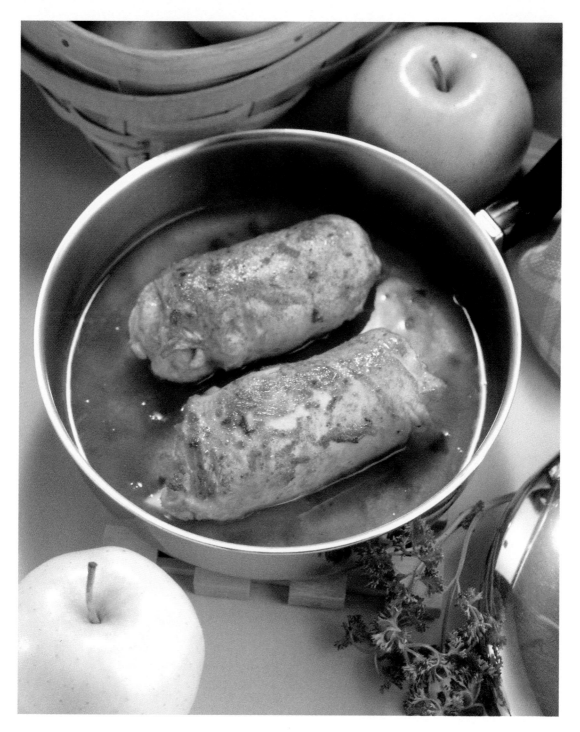

Stuffed Chicken Breasts

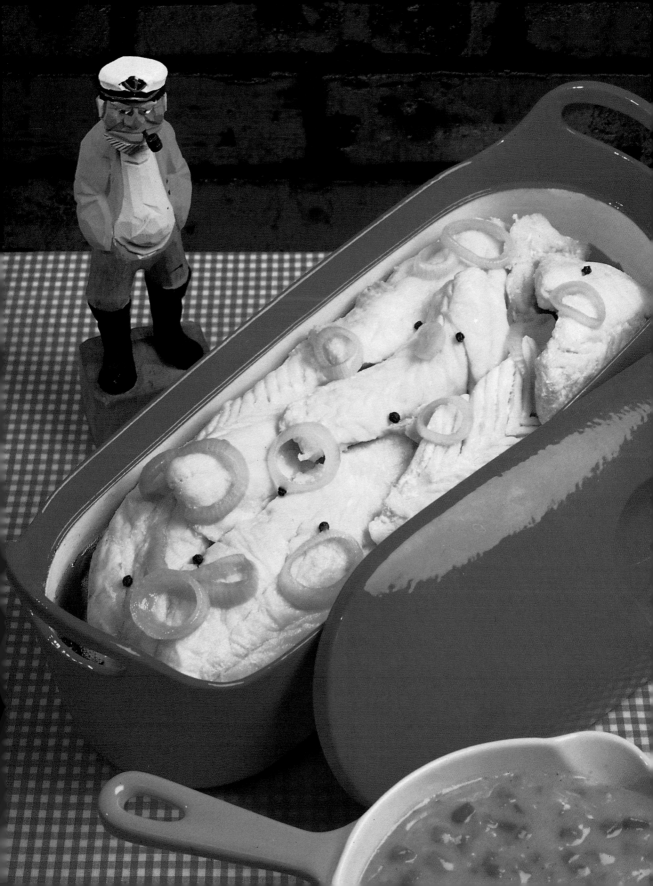

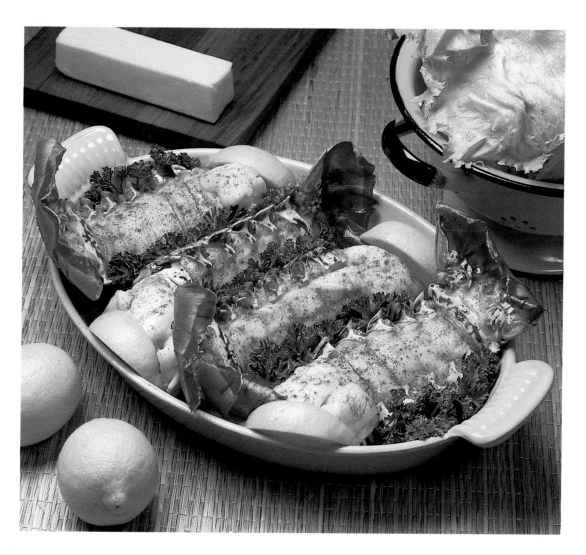

Ale-Poached Fish with Pimiento Sauce (left)

Lettuce Baked Lobster Tails

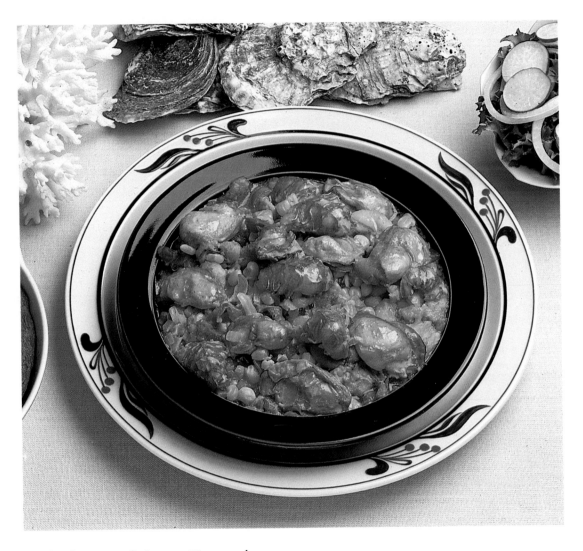

Rock Shrimp and Oyster Manquechon

Creamy Cucumber Soup

FOUR SERVINGS

2 medium cucumbers, peeled and sliced (about 3 cups)
1 cup water
¼ cup onion slices
¼ teaspoon salt substitute
⅛ teaspoon pepper

■ ■ ■

¼ cup all-purpose flour
2 cups unsalted chicken broth, divided
¼ teaspoon ground cloves
¼ teaspoon paprika
1 cup plain lowfat yogurt, chilled
1 tablespoon finely chopped dill

*Exchange Values
Per Serving:*
½ Milk
½ Bread

*100 Calories
(17% from Fat)*
13.8gm Carbohydrates
6.9gm Protein
1.8gm Fat
4mg Cholesterol
431mg Sodium
549mg Potassium

Combine the cucumber slices with water, onion, salt substitute and pepper in a 2 quart saucepan. Cook until very soft, approximately 30 minutes. Put through a strainer or blend in a food processor until smooth. Set aside. Combine the flour with ½ of the chicken broth in the same saucepan. Stir until smooth and gradually add the remaining chicken broth and blend well. Add the cucumber puree, cloves, and paprika. Stir over medium heat until the mixture begins to simmer. Reduce the heat and simmer for an additional 2 minutes. Do not boil. Remove from the heat and refrigerate. Before serving, stir in the yogurt and dill. Serve very cold in chilled bowls. Refreshing!

Fall Harvest Soup

FOUR SERVINGS

1 **2-pound butternut squash, peeled and cubed**
4 **cups chicken broth**
2 **cooking apples, peeled and quartered**
2 **tablespoons lemon juice**
   Pepper to taste
¼ **teaspoon nutmeg**
   Mrs. Dash salt substitute to taste
1 **cup skim milk**

Cook the squash in chicken stock until tender, about 10 minutes. Add the apples and cook until soft. Puree the squash and apples in a food processor. Reheat with the stock, and add the lemon juice and seasonings to taste. Stir in the milk. Heat thoroughly, but do not boil.

Exchange Values
Per Serving:
½ Fruit
2 Bread

200 Calories
(8% from Fat)
39.9gm Carbohydrates
9.3gm Protein
1.9gm Fat
1.3mg Cholesterol
811mg Sodium
1293mg Potassium

Savory Zucchini Soup

FOUR SERVINGS

1¼ **teaspoons Italian seasonings**
1½ **cups chopped onions**
1½ **cups chopped celery**
1½ **tablespoons liquid margarine**
1½ **cups grated unpeeled zucchini**
1½ **cups unsalted chicken broth**

2½ **cups skim milk**
¼ **teaspoon white pepper**
2 **low-sodium chicken bouillon cubes**

Sauté the seasonings, onions, and celery in margarine until transparent. Add the zucchini and chicken broth. Simmer for 10 minutes. Just before serving, add the skim milk, pepper, and bouillon cubes. Heat to serving temperature, but do not boil.

Exchange Values
Per Serving:
½ Milk
2 Vegetable
1 Fat

138 Calories
(32% from Fat)
16.4gm Carbohydrates
7.2gm Protein
5.3gm Fat
1.4mg Cholesterol
166mg Sodium
904mg Potassium

Potato and Leek Soup

SIX SERVINGS

4 leeks
1 medium onion
1 bunch scallions
3 tablespoons liquid margarine
4 cups unsalted chicken broth
5 medium potatoes, peeled and thinly sliced
1 cup skim milk
Fresh chives

*Exchange Values
Per Serving:*
3 Vegetable
2 Bread
1½ Fat

*323 Calories
(19% from Fat)*
58.7gm Carbohydrates
8.2gm Protein
7gm Fat
1.3mg Cholesterol
120mg Sodium
1907mg Potassium

*C*hop the leeks, onion, and scallions, and sauté in the margarine until slightly brown. Add the chicken stock and potatoes, and cook until soft. Puree in a blender. Add the skim milk, and reheat but do not boil. Serve with chopped fresh chives as a garnish.

Hearty Potato Soup

EIGHT SERVINGS

1 medium onion, chopped
⅓ cup chopped green pepper
1 clove garlic, minced
1 tablespoon liquid margarine
■ ■ ■
½ cup chicken broth
2 carrots sliced and diced
¼ cup diced celery
4 small potatoes, pared and diced
Pinch nutmeg
1½ teaspoons curry powder
2½ cups skim milk
Pinch salt and pepper

*Exchange Values
Per Serving:*
½ Milk
½ Vegetable
1 Bread

*116 Calories
(14% from Fat)*
20.2gm Carbohydrates
5.1gm Protein
1.8gm Fat
1.3mg Cholesterol
145mg Sodium
642mg Potassium

*S*auté the onion, green pepper, and garlic in margarine in a saucepan for 3 to 4 minutes. Add the remaining ingredients and stir. Simmer for 35 to 45 minutes or until the potatoes are tender. Pour into a blender and puree. Pour back into the saucepan and warm thoroughly.

Tofu Soup

SIX SERVINGS

8 ounces fresh tofu
½ cup water
1 tablespoon minced dried onion
½ teaspoon low sodium instant chicken bouillon granules
½ teaspoon dried basil, crushed
1 10-ounce package frozen chopped broccoli

▪ ▪ ▪

1 10¾-ounce can condensed cream of potato soup
2 cups skim milk
¾ cup shredded Swiss cheese (reduced sodium, reduced cholesterol)
1 teaspoon parsley flakes

*P*lace the tofu in a double thickness of cheesecloth or paper toweling. Press gently to get as much of the moisture out of the tofu as possible. Cut the tofu into ½-inch cubes. Combine the water, dried onion, bouillon granules, and basil in a saucepan. Bring to a boil. Stir in the frozen broccoli, and return to a boil. Reduce the heat, cover, and simmer for 5 minutes or until tender. Do not drain. Stir in the cream of potato soup. Gradually add the milk and heat almost to a boil. Reduce the heat. Add the tofu and cheese, stirring until the cheese is melted.

Exchange Values Per Serving:
½ Milk
1 Vegetable
3 Meat
1 Fat

374 Calories
(51% from Fat)
18.0gm Carbohydrates
31.9gm Protein
21.1gm Fat
30.3mg Cholesterol
469mg Sodium
350mg Potassium

Zucchini Soup

EIGHT SERVINGS

8 small zucchini, sliced
1 cup water
1 small onion, minced
2 tablespoons reduced sodium chicken bouillon granules
2 teaspoons salt substitute
1 teaspoon fresh parsley

▪ ▪ ▪

¼ cup cornstarch
3 cups skim milk
3 tablespoons cholesterol-free margarine
2 tablespoons low-sodium chicken bouillon granules

Exchange Values Per Serving:
1 Vegetable
½ Milk
1 Fat

99 Calories
(42% from Fat)
10.8gm Carbohydrates
4.2gm Protein
4.6gm Fat
2mg Cholesterol
92mg Sodium
350mg Potassium

*C*ook the zucchini in water with the onion, 2 tablespoons of chicken bouillon, the salt substitute, and parsley in a medium saucepan until tender.

Place the cornstarch in a small bowl. Gradually stir in a small amount of the skim milk, mixing until all of the cornstarch is dissolved. Combine the cornstarch mixture, the remaining milk, margarine, and 2 tablespoons chicken bouillon granules in a saucepan. Simmer over medium heat, stirring occasionally, until the mixture is thickened. Puree the zucchini mixture in a blender, then add it to the thickened mixture in the saucepan. Serve hot.

Tuna Chowder

FOUR SERVINGS

1 10¾-ounce can low-sodium chicken broth
1 cup diced potatoes
1 pound yellowfin tuna steaks, skinned and cubed
½ cup *each* chopped onions, carrots, and celery
½ cup frozen corn
½ teaspoon dried basil
¼ teaspoon dried thyme
½ cup skim milk
1 tablespoon chopped parsley

Exchange Values
Per Serving:
½ Vegetable
1 Bread
3 Meat

245 Calories
(23% from Fat)
16.8gm Carbohydrates
29.6gm Protein
6.3gm Fat
44mg Cholesterol
97mg Sodium
936mg Potassium

*M*ix the chicken broth with 1 soup can of water. Add the potatoes and simmer for 10 to 15 minutes, until tender. Remove the potatoes from the broth, reserving the liquid. Puree the cooked potatoes with ¼ cup of broth. Add the tuna, vegetables, seasonings, and pureed potatoes to the remaining broth in the saucepan. Simmer for 8 to 10 minutes, until the fish flakes easily. Stir in the milk and heat to serving temperature without boiling. Sprinkle with parsley just before serving.

Fall Harvest Chowder

EIGHT SERVINGS

1   large potato, peeled and cubed
¼   cup all-purpose flour
3   tablespoons liquid margarine
4   cups unsalted chicken stock
■ ■ ■
1   large onion, minced
2   ribs celery, minced
1   large carrot, finely chopped
1   tablespoon margarine
½   cup broccoli flowerets
½   cup cauliflower flowerets
■ ■ ■
2   cups skim milk
1   clove garlic, minced
    Pepper to taste

*Exchange Values
Per Serving:*
½ Milk
½ Vegetable
½ Bread
1 Fat

139 Calories
(43% from Fat)
16.2gm Carbohydrates
4.3gm Protein
6.6gm Fat
1mg Cholesterol
109mg Sodium
809mg Potassium

*P*lace the potato in cold water and bring to a boil. Cool and reserve. Melt the margarine in a saucepan, and add the flour slowly to make a roux. Bring the chicken stock to a boil in a stock pot and thicken with the flour and margarine roux. Bring back to a boil, and reduce the heat to a simmer. Sauté the onion, celery, and carrots in margarine for 10 minutes, stirring constantly. Add the vegetables for the last 5 minutes of cooking. Strain the chicken stock into this mixture and add the potatoes. Bring to a boil and simmer until the vegetables are done. Add the skim milk and seasonings, and gently return to just boiling. Serve at once.

Turkey Chowder

FOUR SERVINGS

½   cup chopped onion
1   cup sliced celery
1   garlic clove, minced
2   tablespoons liquid margarine
2   tablespoons all-purpose flour
½   teaspoon salt substitute
¼   teaspoon ground black pepper

*Exchange Values
Per Serving:*
1 Vegetable
1 Bread
2 Meat
1 Fat

5   cups turkey broth
2   potatoes, peeled and cubed
1   cup chopped carrots

      ■ ■ ■

1   cup cooked, chopped turkey

324 Calories
(29% from Fat)
29.9gm Carbohydrates
26.4gm Protein
10.4gm Fat
43mg Cholesterol
1118mg Sodium
1233mg Potassium

Sauté the onion, celery, and garlic in the margarine. Add the flour, salt substitute, and pepper. Gradually add the broth, stirring constantly. Add the potatoes and carrots. Cover and simmer for 15 minutes, or until the vegetables are tender. Add the turkey and continue to cook over low heat for 10 minutes.

This can be served over long grain brown rice.

Clam Chowder

EIGHT SERVINGS

½ cup chopped mushrooms
1   cup chopped celery
1   cup chopped onion
¼ cup cholesterol-free margarine
1   quart boiling water
1   cup finely diced carrots
1   cup diced potatoes

      ■ ■ ■

¼ cup cholesterol-free margarine
¼ cup all-purpose flour
1   gallon skim milk

      ■ ■ ■

2   6½-ounce cans chopped clams, including juice
1   tablespoon chopped pimientos
¼ cup dry white wine

Exchange Values
Per Serving:
2 Milk
½ Vegetable
½ Bread
1 Meat
1 Fat

329 Calories
(29% from Fat)
33.7gm Carbohydrates
25.3gm Protein
10.1gm Fat
36.7mg Cholesterol
394mg Sodium
1246mg Potassium

Sauté the mushrooms, celery, and onion in ¼ cup margarine in a large heavy saucepan. Add the water, carrots, and potatoes. Simmer for 20 minutes, or until the vegetables are tender.

While the vegetables are simmering, make a roux by melting ¼ cup of margarine in a saucepan over medium heat. Stir in the flour and mix well. Add the skim milk and stir occasionally until thickened. Set aside. When the vegetables are tender, add the clams with their juice, the pimientos, and white wine. Add the white sauce. Cook 10 minutes longer. Serve piping hot.

Family Style Chili

1   cup chopped onion
1   cup diced green pepper
2   pounds lean ground chuck
2   tablespoons liquid margarine

2   cloves garlic, minced
3   tablespoons chili powder
1½ teaspoons paprika
3   whole cloves
4   cups cooked, skinned tomatoes

1   15-ounce can kidney beans

*Exchange Values
Per Serving:*
1½ Vegetable
3 Meat
1 Fat
1 Bread

*384 Calories
(36% from Fat)*
19.3gm Carbohydrates
42.5gm Protein
15.4gm Fat
115mg Cholesterol
330mg Sodium
902mg Potassium

*B*rown the onion, green pepper and ground chuck in the margarine. Add the minced garlic, seasonings, and tomatoes. Cover and cook over low heat for about 1 hour. Add the kidney beans during the last 15 minutes of cooking time. This can be served in a bowl as soup or over spaghetti noodles as a main dish.

Hearty Fruit Soup

1   29-ounce can unsweetened pear halves
1   29-ounce can unsweetened sliced peaches
1   cup unsweetened pineapple bits

1½ cups raisins
¼   cup water
½   teaspoon cornstarch
3   tablespoons brown sugar substitute
½   teaspoon grated lemon peel
¼   teaspoon ground allspice
⅛   teaspoon ground cloves
¼   teaspoon cinnamon

*Exchange Values
Per Serving:*
1 Fruit

*45 Calories
(2% from Fat)*
11.7gm Carbohydrates
0.5gm Protein
0.1gm Fat
0mg Cholesterol
3mg Sodium
147mg Potassium

*D*rain the pears, peaches and pineapples, reserving 1½ cups of the mixed juices. Cut the pears into chunks. In a 4-quart saucepan over high heat combine the raisins, water mixed with the cornstarch, brown sugar, lemon peel, allspice, cloves, cinnamon, and reserved fruit juice in a 4-quart saucepan. Bring to a boil, and reduce the heat to a simmer. Cover and simmer for 10 minutes. Add the pears, peaches, and pineapple. Serve hot or cold. One serving equals ⅓ cup.

Pineapple and Peach Soup

EIGHT SERVINGS

1½ **pounds peaches**
½ **a fresh pineapple**
1 **cup fresh orange juice**
1 **cup unsweetened pineapple juice**
2 **cups plain lowfat yogurt**
2 **packets artificial sweetener**
½ **cup dry white wine**
1 **tablespoon lemon juice**
  Lime slices and mint leaves for garnish

Exchange Values
Per Serving:
½ Milk
2 Fruit

142 Calories
(13% from Fat)
28.5gm Carbohydrates
4.1gm Protein
1.3gm Fat
3.5mg Cholesterol
41mg Sodium
480mg Potassium

*P*eel and pit the peaches. Puree the peaches and pineapple in a food processor until smooth. Add the juices, yogurt, sweetener, and wine, and blend well. Put the soup through a fine strainer. Serve chilled, garnished with lime slices and mint leaves.

Refreshing Chilled Strawberry Soup

FOUR SERVINGS

2½ cups strawberry puree, strained
1   cup skim milk
1   cup plain lowfat yogurt
1   package sugar substitute
1   teaspoon Triple sec

Combine the puree, milk, and yogurt in a blender. Add sugar substitute and triple sec to taste. Chill.

Exchange Values Per Serving:
½ Fruit
½ Milk

92 Calories
(14% from Fat)
14.8gm Carbohydrates
5.7gm Protein
1.4gm Fat
5mg Cholesterol
74mg Sodium
421mg Potassium

Summer Strawberry and Burgundy Soup

EIGHT SERVINGS

3   pints strawberries, washed and hulled
1   cup water
    ■ ■ ■
4   packages sugar substitute
¼   cup all-purpose flour
2   cups burgundy
2   cups unsweetened orange juice
    ■ ■ ■
3   cups plain lowfat yogurt
1   cup skim milk
    ■ ■ ■
    Sliced strawberries
    Mint leaves

Exchange Values Per Serving:
½ Milk
1 Fruit
½ Bread
½ Fat

185 Calories
(9% from Fat)
26.3gm Carbohydrates
7.1gm Protein
1.9gm Fat
5.8mg Cholesterol
81mg Sodium
627mg Potassium

Quarter the strawberries and cook in water for 10 minutes. In a separate saucepan, combine the sugar substitute and flour. Stir in the wine and orange juice. Heat, stirring constantly until the mixture boils, approximately 10 minutes. Remove from the heat immediately and add the strawberries and cool. Puree in a blender or food processor and add the yogurt and skim milk. Chill. Serve garnished with strawberries and mint leaves.

Whole Wheat Bread

THIRTY SERVINGS

2 cups lowfat milk
½ cup sugar
1 cup cholesterol-free oil
1½ teaspoons salt substitute
2 cups hot water

■ ■ ■

4 egg whites
4 tablespoons dry yeast
10 cups whole wheat flour
6 cups all-purpose flour

*Exchange Values
Per Serving:*
3 Bread
1½ Fat

317 Calories
(24% from Fat)
52gm Carbohydrates
9.3gm Protein
8.8gm Fat
19.5mg Cholesterol
15mg Sodium
345mg Potassium

Scald the milk and pour into a bowl with the sugar, oil, and salt substitute. Add the hot water. Cool until lukewarm.

To the cooled mixture add the eggs, yeast, and 4 cups of whole wheat flour, and mix with a whisk. Add the remaining whole wheat and all-purpose flour. Turn out onto a floured surface and knead until elastic and smooth. Place in an oiled bowl and let rise until double in bulk. Punch down and knead again. Form into loaves and/ or rolls and let rise until double. Bake at 375° for 15 to 25 minutes, until brown and sounds hollow when tapped on top. Remove from the pan immediately and cool on a wire rack.

Blackberry and Zucchini Bread

FIFTEEN SERVINGS

¼ cup oil
½ cup sugar
3 egg whites
1 tablespoon freshly grated orange rind
½ cup orange juice
1½ cups whole wheat flour
1½ cups all-purpose flour
1 teaspoon baking soda
2 teaspoons baking powder
1 16-ounce can of blackberries packed in water, drained
1½ cups finely shredded zucchini

Combine all ingredients except berries and zucchini until just blended. Fold in the berries and zucchini. Turn into a sprayed loaf pan and bake at 350° for 1½ hours. Check after the first 45 minutes to prevent browning too quickly.

Exchange Values Per Serving:
½ Fruit
1 Fat
1 Bread

172 Calories
(21% from Fat)
31gm Carbohydrates
4.3gm Protein
4.1gm Fat
0mg Cholesterol
112mg Sodium
189mg Potassium

Pumpkin-Apple Bread

FIFTEEN SERVINGS

⅓ cup cholesterol-free oil
2 tablespoons sugar
2 egg whites
¾ cup canned pumpkin

■ ■ ■

2 cups all-purpose flour
1 tablespoon baking powder
½ teaspoon baking soda
1 teaspoon cinnamon

■ ■ ■

½ cup orange juice
2 large apples, peeled, cored, and cubed

Exchange Values Per Serving:
¼ Fruit
1 Bread
1 Fat

134 Calories
(36% from Fat)
19.2gm Carbohydrates
2.4gm Protein
5.4gm Fat

Beat together the oil, sugar, egg, and pumpkin until light and fluffy.

Combine the flour, baking powder, baking soda, and cinnamon in a bowl. Stir in the pumpkin mixture and the orange juice. Stir in the apple chunks. Pour into an oiled loaf pan. Bake at 350° for 40 to 45 minutes. Cool on a wire rack.

0mg Cholesterol
101mg Sodium
84mg Potassium

Oat Bran Bread

THIRTY SERVINGS

2½ cups boiling water
½   cup cholesterol-free margarine
¼   cup honey
■ ■ ■
2   ¼-ounce packages active dry yeast
1¾ cups oat bran
1   cup chopped nuts
■ ■ ■
2   eggs
6   cups whole wheat flour

*Exchange Values
Per Serving:*
1½ Bread
1 Fat

168 Calories
(35% from Fat)
23.8gm Carbohydrates
4.3gm Protein
6.7gm Fat
15.7mg Cholesterol
35mg Sodium
73mg Potassium

Combine the boiling water, margarine, and honey in a bowl. Cool to lukewarm. Combine the yeast with the oat bran and nuts, and mix well. Whisk into the lukewarm liquid. Add the eggs and mix well. Add the flour, and mix well by hand. This will make a stiff dough. Turn out onto a floured surface and knead for approximately 10 minutes or until smooth in texture. Place in an oiled bowl, cover, and let rise until double in bulk, approximately 1 hour. Punch down and form into 2 loaves. Place in loaf pans and allow to double in size. Bake at 375° for 30 to 35 minutes or until golden brown. Cool for at least 1 hour before slicing.

Makes 2 loaves, or 30 servings.

Banana Bread

FIFTEEN SERVINGS

2   cups all-purpose flour
2   teaspoons baking powder
½   teaspoon baking soda
½   teaspoon cinnamon
1½ cups sliced bananas (2 large bananas)
1   egg
½   cup vegetable oil
2   tablespoons sugar
½   cup orange juice

*Exchange Values
Per Serving:*
½ Fruit
1 Bread
1½ Fat

*155 Calories
(45% from Fat)*
19gm Carbohydrates
2.4gm Protein
7.9gm Fat
18.3mg Cholesterol
78mg Sodium
100mg Potassium

Combine the flour, baking powder, baking soda, and cinnamon. Stir to blend. Puree the bananas. Add the bananas and remaining ingredients and mix well. Pour into an oiled loaf pan. Bake at 350° for 40 to 50 minutes. Cool on a wire rack.

Golden Apple Wheat Loaf

FIFTEEN SERVINGS

1½ cups chopped Golden Delicious apples
¼   cup sugar
1   tablespoon brown sugar
1   teaspoon baking soda
1   teaspoon Puritan oil
1   cup sugar-free lemon-lime soda
4   egg whites, slightly beaten
1½ cups all-purpose flour
2½ teaspoons baking powder
1   cup whole wheat flour
1   cup chopped walnuts

*Exchange Values
Per Serving:*
1 Bread
1 Fat
¼ Fruit

*156 Calories
(29% from Fat)*
24gm Carbohydrates
4.4gm Protein
5.2gm Fat
0mg Cholesterol
130mg Sodium
113mg Potassium

Combine the apples, fructose, brown sugar, baking soda, and oil in a large bowl. Add the lemon-lime soda and mix. Add the egg whites. Sift the flour and baking powder together into a separate bowl. Stir in the whole wheat flour. Add the apple mixture and mix well. Fold in the walnuts. Turn into a greased 9x5-inch loaf pan. Bake at 350° for 1 hour or until the bread tests done.

Apple-Raisin Muffins

TWELVE MUFFINS

2 cups all-purpose flour
2 teaspoons baking powder
½ teaspoon baking soda
1 teaspoon cinnamon
1 tablespoon sugar
1 egg
3 tablespoons liquid oil
½ cup unsweetened apple juice
1 cup unsweetened applesauce
⅓ cup raisins
½ cup chopped walnuts

*Exchange Values
Per Muffin:*
½ Fruit
1 Bread
1½ Fat

168 Calories
(35% from Fat)
236gm Carbohydrates
3.6gm Protein
7.2gm Fat
22.8mg Cholesterol
99mg Sodium
108mg Potassium

Combine all of the ingredients, mixing until just blended. Pour into prepared muffin tins. Bake at 350° for 20 minutes.

Blueberry Banana Muffins

TWELVE MUFFINS

1 cup whole wheat flour
1 cup all-purpose flour
1 teaspoon baking soda
2 teaspoons baking powder
½ teaspoon cinnamon
½ cup rolled oats
¼ cup cholesterol-free oil
4 tablespoons sugar
2 egg whites
1 tablespoon lemon juice
½ cup 100% pure unsweetened orange juice
1 cup fozen blueberries
2 whole bananas, mashed

*Exchange Values
Per Muffin:*
½ Fruit
1 Bread
1 Fat

171 Calories
(27% from Fat)
28.7gm Carbohydrates
3.5gm Protein
5.2gm Fat
0mg Cholesterol
130mg Sodium
170mg Potassium

Combine all of the ingredients except the berries and bananas until just blended. Gently add the berries and bananas by hand with a wooden spoon. Spoon into prepared muffin tins. Bake at 350° for 20 minutes.

Apricot-Oat Bran Muffins

2 cups oat bran cereal
¼ cup Millers bran
½ cup whole wheat flour
2½ teaspoons baking powder
½ teaspoon cinnamon
½ cup diced dried apricots
4 egg whites
½ cup skim milk
1 tablespoon oil
⅓ cup honey

■ ■ ■

1 cup all-purpose flour
¼ cup liquid margarine
3 tablespoons whole rolled oats
½ teaspoon cinnamon

*Exchange Values
Per Muffin:*
2 Bread
1 Fat

183 Calories
(28% from Fat)
29gm Carbohydrates
6.3gm Protein
6gm Fat
0mg Cholesterol
153mg Sodium
179mg Potassium

Combine the brans, whole wheat flour, baking powder, cinnamon, and apricots. Add the egg whites, milk, oil, and honey, stirring until just blended. Pour into prepared muffin tins.

Combine the all-purpose flour, margarine, oats, and cinnamon, and sprinkle over the batter. Bake at 350° for 15 to 20 minutes.

Banana Muffins

2 cups flour (whole wheat, unbleached, or combination)
2 teaspoons baking bowder
½ teaspoon baking soda
½ teaspoon cinnamon

■ ■ ■

1 egg or egg substitute
1 teaspoon vanilla extract
2 tablespoons oil
2 tablespoons sugar
¼ cup orange juice
¼ cup water
2 large bananas, mashed

■ ■ ■

*Exchange Values
Per Muffin:*
½ Fruit
1 Bread
1 Fat

126 Calories
(34% from Fat)
19.2gm Carbohydrates
2.7gm Protein
4.7gm Fat
15mg Cholesterol
88mg Sodium
110mg Potassium

½ cup all-purpose flour
3 tablespoons liquid margarine
¼ teaspoon cinnamon

Combine 2 cups of flour, the baking powder, baking soda, and ½ teaspoon of cinnamon in a mixing bowl. Stir to blend. Pour the egg, vanilla, oil, sugar, orange juice, water, and bananas into a separate bowl, and blend until smooth. Pour the banana mixture into the dry ingredients and stir until just blended. Pour into a well-sprayed muffin pan.

Combine ½ cup of flour, the margarine, and ¼ teaspoon of cinnamon, and sprinkle over the muffins. Bake at 350° for 15 minutes.

Blueberry Muffins

TWELVE MUFFINS

½ cup all-purpose flour
½ cup whole wheat flour
2 teaspoons baking powder
1 teaspoon baking soda
3 tablespoons sugar
1 teaspoon cinnamon
   ■ ■ ■
2 egg whites
1½ cups skim milk
3 tablespoons oil
   ■ ■ ■
1 cup frozen blueberries
   ■ ■ ■
½ cup all-purpose flour
½ cup liquid margarine
1½ teaspoons cinnamon

*Exchange Values
Per Muffin:*
2 Bread
2 Fat

237 Calories
(43% from Fat)
28.6gm Carbohydrates
5.1gm Protein
11.9gm Fat
2.3mg Cholesterol
217mg Sodium
113mg Potassium

Combine ½ cup of all-purpose flour with the whole wheat flour in a large bowl. Add the baking powder, baking soda, sugar and 1 teaspoon of cinnamon. Combine the egg whites, milk, and oil in a separate bowl. Make a well in the center of the dry ingredients, and add the egg mixture. Stir until just combined. Fold in the blueberries carefully with a wooden spoon. Pour into muffin tins. Combine ½ cup of all-purpose flour with the margarine and 1½ teaspoons of cinnamon. Sprinkle over the muffins. Bake at 400° for 20 to 25 minutes.

Carrot Cake Muffins

TWELVE MUFFINS

1½ cups whole wheat flour
1   teaspoon baking soda
1   tablespoon baking powder
1   teaspoon ground cinnamon
1   egg
2   tablespoons vegetable oil
¼   cup raisins
¼   cup chopped walnuts
½   cup orange juice
1   8-ounce can unsweetened crushed pineapple, undrained
1½ cups grated carrots

Exchange Values
Per Muffin:
½ Fruit
1 Bread
1 Fat

125 Calories
(32% from Fat)
19.2gm Carbohydrates
3.3gm Protein
4.6gm Fat
22.8mg Cholesterol
165mg Sodium
186mg Potassium

Combine the flour, baking soda, baking powder, and cinnamon in a bowl. Add the remaining ingredients and stir to blend. Spoon into oiled muffin tins or paper muffin cups. Bake at 350° for 20 to 25 minutes.

Cranberry-Orange Muffins

TWELVE MUFFINS

½ cup fresh or frozen cranberries
1   egg
½   cup orange juice
1   tablespoon vegetable oil
1   teaspoon grated orange rind
1   cup all-purpose flour
2   teaspoons baking powder
½   teaspoon baking soda
1   tablespoon sugar
1   teaspoon vanilla extract
¼   cup chopped walnuts

Exchange Values
Per Muffin:
1 Bread
½ Fat

79 Calories
(36% from Fat)
10.7gm Carbohydrates
1.9gm Protein
3.2gm Fat
20mg Cholesterol
90mg Sodium
49mg Potassium

Combine all of the ingredients, stirring until just blended. Pour into prepared muffin tins. Bake at 350° for 20 minutes.

Oat Bran Muffins

SIX MUFFINS

¾ cup whole wheat flour
¾ cup oat bran cereal
2 tablespoons baking powder
½ teaspoon cinnamon
3 tablespoons oil
3 tablespoons honey
¾ cup orange juice

Exchange Values
Per Muffin:
2 Bread
1 Fat

175 Calories
(38% from Fat)
27.2gm Carbohydrates
2.8gm Protein
7.3gm Fat
0mg Cholesterol
340mg Sodium
152mg Potassium

Combine the dry ingredients in a large bowl. Mix the oil, syrup, and orange juice. Make a well in the center of the dry ingredients and add the oil mixture. Stir until blended. Fill 6 oiled muffin tins ¾ full. Bake at 375° for 15 minutes.

Oat Bran-Banana Muffins

THIRTY-SIX MUFFINS

4 cups whole wheat flour
4 cups all purpose flour
2 cups Millers bran
4 cups rolled oats
2 tablespoons baking powder
2 teaspoons baking soda
2 teaspoons cinnamon
¼ teaspoon nutmeg
4 tablespoons brown sugar
4 eggs
½ cup oil
2 cups unsweetened orange juice
4 small bananas
1 cup toasted unsalted sunflower seeds

Exchange Values
Per Muffin:
½ Fruit
2 Bread
1 Fat

213 Calories
(25% from Fat)
34.4gm Carbohydrates
6.8gm Protein
6.8gm Fat
30.4mg Cholesterol
137mg Sodium
264mg Potassium

Combine all of the ingredients, stirring until blended. Pour into prepared muffin tins. Bake at 350° for 20 minutes.

Oatmeal-Banana Muffins

TWELVE MUFFINS

3 cups all-purpose flour
¾ cup rolled oats
1 tablespoon baking powder
½ teaspoon cinnamon
1 tablespoon sugar
1 egg
2 tablespoons vegetable oil
1 cup unsweetened orange juice
2 small bananas, chopped

Combine the flour, oats, baking powder, cinnamon, and sugar in a bowl. Add the remaining ingredients. Stir until blended. Spoon into oiled muffin tins or paper muffin cups. Bake at 375° for 15 to 30 minutes.

*Exchange Values
Per Muffin:*
½ Fruit
2 Bread
1 Fat

182 Calories
(17% from Fat)
32.7gm Carbohydrates
4.8gm Protein
3.4gm Fat
22.8mg Cholesterol
91mg Sodium
134mg Potassium

Pumpkin-Apple Bran Muffins

EIGHTEEN MUFFINS

1 cup all-purpose flour
½ cup bran
1 teaspoon sugar
2 teaspoons baking powder
½ teaspoon cinnamon
2 tablespoons vegetable oil
½ cup canned pumpkin
2 egg whites
¾ cup orange juice
½ cup chopped apple

■ ■ ■

1 cup wheat germ
½ cup all-purpose flour
4 tablespoons margarine

Combine 1 cup of flour, the bran, sugar, baking powder, and cinnamon in a large bowl. Add the oil, pumpkin, egg whites, orange juice, and apple, stirring until just blended. Spoon into sprayed or paper-lined muffin tins.

*Exchange Values
Per Muffin:*
1 Bread
1 Fat

109 Calories
(42% from Fat)
14.1gm Carbohydrates
3.7gm Protein
5.1gm Fat
0mg Cholesterol
77mg Sodium
125mg Potassium

Combine the wheat germ, ½ cup of flour, and the butter until the mixture resembles coarse crumbs. Sprinkle over the muffins. Bake at 350° for 15 to 20 minutes.

Buttermilk Biscuits

TWENTY-SIX BISCUITS

4 cups all-purpose flour
2 tablespoons baking powder
1 teaspoon salt substitute
½ cup margarine
1 pint buttermilk

Stir together the flour, baking powder, and salt substitute in a large mixing bowl. Cut in the margarine until coarse, and gradually pour in the buttermilk. Stir, then knead quickly to make a stiff dough. Do not overwork. Roll out to ½-inch thickness and cut into biscuits of the desired size. Bake at 375° for 18 minutes, and serve immediately.

The dough can be kept in the refrigerator for up to 6 hours after being cut.

*Exchange Values
Per Biscuit:*
1 Bread
1 Fat

*104 Calories
(32% from Fat)*
14.6gm Carbohydrates
2.5gm Protein
3.8gm Fat
0.5mg Cholesterol
130mg Sodium
103mg Potassium

Yogurt Drop Biscuits

SIXTEEN BISCUITS

1 tablespoon baking powder
¾ teaspoon salt substitute
2 cups sifted all-purpose flour
¼ cup plain lowfat yogurt
1 cup skim milk

Sift together the dry ingredients. Stir in the yogurt and skim milk. Drop the batter into well-sprayed muffin tins, filling them one third full. The batter will be very soft. Bake at 425° for about 10 minutes. The batter can be made ahead of time and refrigerated until needed.

*Exchange Values
Per Biscuit:*
1 Bread

*65 Calories
(3% from Fat)*
13.1gm Carbohydrates
2.3gm Protein
0.2gm Fat
0.5mg Cholesterol
74mg Sodium
167mg Potassium

Whole Wheat and Yogurt Biscuits

TWELVE BISCUITS

2 cups whole wheat flour
2 teaspoons baking powder
⅓ teaspoon salt substitute
3 tablespoons safflower oil
¼ cup skim milk
¼ cup plain lowfat yogurt

*S*ift together the dry ingredients. Mix in the safflower oil and work by hand until of the consistency of coarse meal. Add the milk and yogurt, and work into a dough. Place on a lightly floured board and roll to ½-inch thickness. Cut with a biscuit cutter. Place the biscuits on a lightly sprayed cookie sheet. Bake at 400° for 10 minutes or until golden brown.

Exchange Values Per Biscuit:
1 Bread
1 Fat

105 Calories
(32% from Fat)
15.3gm Carbohydrates
2.4gm Protein
3.7gm Fat
0.2mg Cholesterol
56mg Sodium
126mg Potassium

Cinnamon French Toast

FOUR SERVINGS

8 slices day-old reduced calorie white bread (40 calories/slice)
8 egg whites
½ cup skim milk
1 teaspoon vanilla extract
½ teaspoon cinnamon
4 teaspoons margarine

*L*ightly beat together the egg whites, skim milk, vanilla, and cinnamon. Heat a griddle and lightly grease with margarine. Coat both sides of the bread with the egg white mixture. Cook until brown and crisp.

Exchange Values Per Serving:
1 Bread
1 Meat
1 Fat

148 Calories
(29% from Fat)
15.5gm Carbohydrates
9.8gm Protein
4.7gm Fat
0.5mg Cholesterol
277mg Sodium
166mg Potassium

Scottish Oat Cakes

TWENTY-FOUR CAKES

4   cups rolled oats
¾   cup all-purpose flour
1½ teaspoons baking powder
½   cup margarine
2   tablespoons skim milk

*P*rocess the oats in a food processor until fine. Combine with the remaining ingredients to form a stiff dough. Let the dough rest for 30 minutes. Roll out to ¼-inch thickness on a floured surface and cut into circles. Bake at 350° for 8 to 10 minutes or until golden brown.

Exchange Values
Per Cake:
1 Bread
1 Fat

100 Calories
(42% from Fat)
11.9gm Carbohydrates
2.7gm Protein
4.7gm Fat
0.1mg Cholesterol
57mg Sodium
58mg Potassium

Scottish Oat-Bran Toast

TWENTY-FOUR CIRCLES

4   cups rolled oats
1   cup Millers bran
¾   cup all-purpose flour
½   teaspoon cinnamon
½   teaspoon vanilla extract
1½ teaspoons baking powder
½   cup margarine
2   tablespoons skim milk

*P*rocess the oats in a food processor until fine. Combine with the remaining ingredients to form a stiff dough. Let the dough rest for 30 minutes. Roll out to ¼-inch thickness on a floured surface. Cut into circles. Bake at 400° for 4 to 8 minutes or until golden.

Exchange Values
Per Circle:
1 Bread
1 Fat

107 Calories
(40% from Fat)
14.0gm Carbohydrates
3.0gm Protein
4.8gm Fat
0.1mg Cholesterol
83mg Sodium
90mg Potassium

Buckwheat Buttermilk Pancakes

SIX PANCAKES

1   egg white
½   cup buttermilk
1   tablespoon vegetable oil
1¼ cups buckwheat flour
1   teaspoon sugar
1   teaspoon baking powder
½   teaspoon baking soda

*B*eat together the egg white, buttermilk, and oil. Add the flour, sugar, baking powder, and baking soda. Stir until the ingredients are just blended. Pour the batter onto a lightly oiled griddle. Cook until bubbles form on the surface and the edges become dry. Turn and cook until golden brown.

Exchange Values
Per Pancake:
1 Bread
1 Fat

105 Calories
(23% from Fat)
18.1gm Carbohydrates
2.5gm Protein
2.7gm Fat
0.4mg Cholesterol
148mg Sodium
105mg Potassium

Buckwheat and Yogurt Pancakes

TWELVE PANCAKES

2   cups buckwheat flour
¾   teaspoon salt substitute
1   teaspoon baking soda
1½ cups lowfat buttermilk
½   cup yogurt
1   egg, beaten
1   teaspoon maple flavoring
1   tablespoon safflower oil

*C*ombine the flour, salt substitute, and soda. Add the remaining ingredients. Pour on a hot, lightly oiled griddle and cook until brown, turning once. Serve hot.

Exchange Values
Per Pancake:
1 Bread
½ Fat

92 Calories
(21% from Fat)
15.2gm Carbohydrates
3.0gm Protein
2.3gm Fat
25mg Cholesterol
113mg Sodium
212mg Potassium

Cornmeal Griddle Cakes

TWELVE PANCAKES

1 cup cornmeal
1 cup all-purpose flour
1 teaspoon salt substitute
1⅓ tablespoons baking powder
1 beaten egg or egg substitute
1½ cups lowfat buttermilk
½ cup yogurt
3 tablespoons safflower oil

Exchange Values
Per Pancake:
1 Bread
1 Fat

128 Calories
(32% from Fat)
17.8gm Carbohydrates
3.8gm Protein
4.5gm Fat
21mg Cholesterol
144mg Sodium
205mg Potassium

*M*ix the dry ingredients in a large bowl. Combine the egg and milk in a small bowl, add the yogurt and whip. Add the milk mixture to the dry ingredients and stir to make a smooth batter. Stir in the safflower oil. Bake on a hot oiled griddle, turning when the underside is browned and the batter is bubbly.

Old-Fashioned Corncakes

THREE SERVINGS

1½ cups lowfat buttermilk
1 tablespoon safflower oil
1 teaspoon baking soda
1 egg white
1 teaspoon salt substitute
¾ cup cornmeal
¼ cup all-purpose flour

Exchange Values
Per Serving:
½ Milk
2 Bread
1 Fat

243 Calories
(22% from Fat)
37.2gm Carbohydrates
8.7gm Protein
6.1gm Fat
3.4mg Cholesterol
419mg Sodium
646mg Potassium

*C*ombine all of the ingredients and mix well. Drop by heaping tablespoons onto a hot griddle. Cook until golden on each side.

Apple Bread Dressing

TEN SERVINGS

4 cups bread crumbs
1 cup chopped celery
1 small onion
1 tablespoon chopped fresh parsley
1 garlic clove, minced
1 cup turkey broth
2 apples, peeled, cored, and diced
¼ teaspoon ground black pepper
¼ teaspoon ground sage
¼ teaspoon dried marjoram
¼ teaspoon diced thyme
⅛ teaspoon dried basil

Exchange Values
Per Serving:
1 Bread

75 Calories
(11% from Fat)
14.7gm Carbohydrates
2.3gm Protein
0.9gm Fat
0.1mg Cholesterol
180mg Sodium
122mg Potassium

Combine all of the ingredients in a bowl. Stir with a wooden spoon. Pour into a lightly oiled casserole pan. Bake at 350° for 35 to 40 minutes. Use to stuff turkey, chicken, or Cornish hens.

Mushroom Dressing

FOUR SERVINGS

2 pounds medium white mushrooms, sliced
4 teaspoons safflower oil
1 cup red wine vinegar
2 teaspoons pepper
8 cloves garlic, finely chopped
2 teaspoons Mrs. Dash of choice

Exchange Values
Per Serving:
3 Vegetable:
1 Fat

116 Calories
(43% from Fat)
16.2gm Carbohydrates
5.2gm Protein
5.5gm Fat
0mg Cholesterol
2mg Sodium
886mg Potassium

Combine all of the ingredients in a large bowl. Cover and refrigerate for 3 days. Stir occasionally. Remove from the refrigerator several hours before serving. Stir well.

Chicken-Apple Dressing

SIX SERVINGS

2 tablespoons cholesterol-free margarine
¼ cup chopped onion
½ cup chopped celery
8 slices day-old or toasted bread, cubed
1 teaspoon sage
½ teaspoon salt substitute
¼ teaspoon pepper
½ cup cubed chicken
½ to ¾ cup chicken broth
½ cup egg substitute equivalent to 2 eggs
1 cup diced peeled apples

Exchange Values
Per Serving:
1½ Bread
1 Meat
1 Fat

215 Calories
(34% from Fat)
24.4gm Carbohydrates
10.8gm Protein
8.1gm Fat
17mg Cholesterol
270mg Sodium
362mg Potassium

*M*elt the margarine in a skillet and sauté the onion and celery until tender. Combine with the bread crumbs in a large bowl. Add the seasonings and cubed chicken. Moisten with chicken broth as desired. Stir in the egg substitute and apples. Bake at 350° for 30 to 40 minutes, or stuff poultry and bake accordingly.

Southern Corn Bread Stuffing

FOUR SERVINGS

3 cups crumbled corn bread
1 cup bread crumbs, cubed
2 cups chicken broth
3 stalks celery, finely chopped
1 large onion, finely chopped
2 egg whites
   Pepper
½ teaspoon sage
½ teaspoon paprika
2 tablespoons liquid margarine

Exchange Values
Per Serving:
1 Bread
½ Meat
1½ Fat

150 Calories
(41% from Fat)
17.4gm Carbohydrates
4.9gm Protein
6.75gm Fat
30.9mg Cholesterol
431mg Sodium
198mg Potassium

*C*ombine all of the ingredients. Turn into a sprayed prepared baking dish and dot the top with margarine. Cover and bake at 350° for 30 minutes. Remove the cover and cook 15 minutes longer.

Baked Grilled Cheese Sandwich

MAKES TWO SANDWICHES

2 egg whites
2 tablespoons skim milk
2 dashes of paprika
4 slices oat brand bread
4 slices low cholesterol cheese (1 ounce each)
   Kosher dill pickle, thinly sliced

*M*ix in a shallow bowl the egg whites, skim milk, and paprika. Dip each side of the bread in the egg mixture and place on a baking sheet that has been sprayed with vegetable spray. Bake in a 400° oven until toasted. Brown on both sides. When golden brown top with cheese and allow to melt slightly. Place on serving plates and top with kosher dill pickle slices.

Exchange Values
Per Serving:
2 Bread
2 Meat

281 Calories
(34% from Fat)
25.5gm Carbohydrates
23gm Protein
10.5gm Fat
35mg Cholesterol
1020mg Sodium
310mg Potassium

Entrees

Baked Chicken and Rice

8 split chicken breasts, skinned and boned (4 ounces each)
¼ cup liquid margarine
1 medium onion, chopped
1 10¾ ounce can cream of chicken soup, undiluted
⅔ cup dry white wine
1 tablespoon parsley, chopped
1 teaspoon paprika
   Pepper to taste
1 tablespoon soy sauce
1 tablespoon lemon juice

Exchange Values
Per Serving:
3 Meat
1 Fat

237 Calories
(36% from Fat)
5.2gm Carbohydrates
28.3gm Protein
9.5gm Fat
70mg Cholesterol
539mg Sodium
388mg Potassium

*L*ightly brown the chicken breasts in margarine in a covered skillet. Remove the chicken from the skillet and place in a medium-size baking dish. Add the onions to the margarine remaining in the skillet, and cook until tender, being careful not to brown. Add the soup, white wine, seasonings and lemon juice. Blend thoroughly and pour over the chicken. Bake at 350° for about 45 minutes. Remove from the oven. Place the chicken on a bed of hot rice (not included in analysis).

Apricot Chicken

6 split chicken breasts, skinned and boned (4 ounces each)
¼ cup liquid margarine
2 teaspoons Mrs. Dash seasoned salt substitute
1 teaspoon garlic powder
½ cup unsweetened pure apricot preserves

*P*lace the chicken breasts in a baking dish and brush with melted margarine. Sprinkle with seasoned salt substitute and garlic powder. Cover and bake at 350° for 45 minutes. Drain the excess fat and juice from the chicken and brush the apricot jam on each piece of chicken with a pastry brush. Return to the oven and bake an additional 15 minutes.

Exchange Values Per Serving:
3 Meat
1 Fat
½ Fruit

288 Calories
(33% from Fat)
19.8gm Carbohydrates
27.2gm Protein
10.7gm Fat
73mg Cholesterol
142mg Sodium
270mg Potassium

Cheese and Sesame Chicken

8 4-ounce boneless and skinless chicken breast fillets
1 cup milk
1 cup crushed cheese crackers
2 tablespoons sesame seeds
   Paprika, garlic powder to taste
1 tablespoon liquid margarine

*S*oak the chicken in milk. Roll in cracker crumbs and place in a baking dish. Sprinkle with sesame seeds. Sprinkle with paprika and garlic powder to taste, and drizzle with margarine. Cover and bake at 350° for 30 to 45 minutes, until tender and the juices run clear. Uncover for the last 5 to 10 minutes to give a crusty topping.

Exchange Values Per Serving:
½ Bread
3 Meat
½ Fat

204 Calories
(20% from Fat)
9.8gm Carbohydrates
29.2gm Protein
4.5gm Fat
68mg Cholesterol
186mg Sodium
364mg Potassium

Baked Fried Chicken

4   split skinless chicken breasts (5 ounces each with bone)
½   cup milk
4   teaspoons margarine
1½ cups Rice Krispies, slightly crushed
    Paprika

Exchange Values
Per Serving:
½ Bread
3 Meat
1 Fat

208 Calories
(23% from Fat)
10.0gm Carbohydrates
28.2gm Protein
5.3gm Fat
68mg Cholesterol
247mg Sodium
333mg Potassium

*W*ash the chicken breasts with water and then cover with milk. Melt the margarine and pour over the Rice Krispies. Drain the chicken and roll in the cereal. Place on an oiled baking sheet and sprinkle with paprika. Bake at 350° for 40 minutes.

Chicken à l'Orange

1   large baking chicken
⅛   teaspoon pepper
1   teaspoon ginger
1   orange, including rind, sliced

1   cup unsweetened orange juice
2   tablespoons honey

    Rinds of 2 oranges, slivered
1   tablespoon all-purpose flour
    Orange slices and parsley for garnish

Exchange Values
Per Serving:
½ Fruit
2 Meat

119 Calories
(17% from Fat)
8.6gm Carbohydrates
15.5gm Protein
2.2gm Fat
50mg Cholesterol
56mg Sodium
228mg Potassium

*R*ub the body of the chicken with the pepper, ginger, and orange slices. Combine the orange juice and honey. Place the chicken in a baking dish and with a pastry brush, brush the skin with the orange juice and honey mixture. Cover and cook at 350° for 1½ to 2 hours. When done, remove the chicken from the pan and pour the juices into a saucepan. Add the slivered orange rinds and flour, and cook until thickened. Serve 2 tablespoons of the sauce over each piece of chicken.

Chicken Popovers

SIX SERVINGS

2   egg whites
1   cup skim milk
1   cup all-purpose flour
2   tablespoons corn oil margarine

■ ■ ■

1½ cups finely chopped chicken
½   cup finely chopped celery
¼   cup reduced calorie mayonnaise
2   tablespoons Italian dressing
1   teaspoon prepared mustard
2   green onions, finely chopped
    Mrs. Dash seasoning
    Paprika

Exchange Values Per Serving:
1 Bread
2 Meat
1 Fat

256 Calories
(34% from Fat)
18.2gm Carbohydrates
22.2gm Protein
9.7gm Fat
53mg Cholesterol
251mg Sodium
282mg Potassium

*B*eat together the egg white, milk, flour and margarine. Pour into a well-greased deep muffin or popover pan, filling the cups ⅔-full. Bake in a preheated 375° oven for 20 to 25 minutes. Do not open the oven while cooking or these will collapse.

Combine the chicken, celery, mayonnaise, dressing, mustard, and onion. Stir well. Sprinkle with Mrs. Dash and paprika to taste. Open each popover and stuff with the chicken mixture.

Chicken Rosemary

FOUR SERVINGS

4   split, skinned boneless chicken breasts (4 ounces each)
4   teaspoons margarine, melted
½   cup all-purpose flour
1   teaspoon crushed rosemary leaves

Exchange Values Per Serving:
1 Bread
3 Meat

215 Calories
(23% from Fat)
11.1gm Carbohydrates
28.4gm Protein
5.4gm Fat
67mg Cholesterol
113mg Sodium
317mg Potassium

*D*ip each piece of chicken in melted margarine, then roll in flour. Place in a shallow greased pan. Sprinkle lightly with rosemary leaves. Add a small amount of water to cover the bottom of the pan. Cover with foil and bake at 350° for about 1 hour. Remove the foil and place under the broiler for a few seconds to brown the chicken.

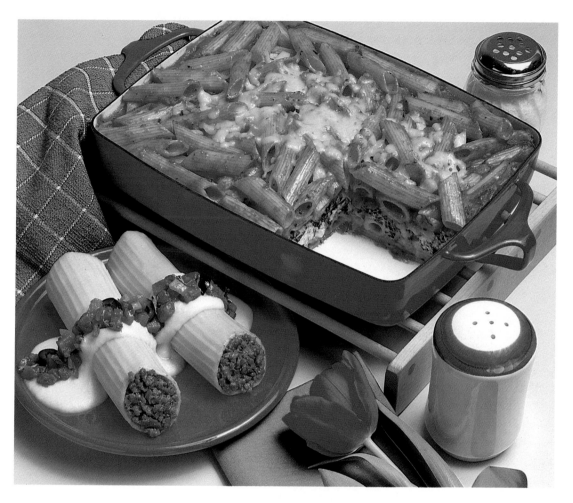

Mostaccioli al Forno / Manicotti with Eggplant Tomato Relish

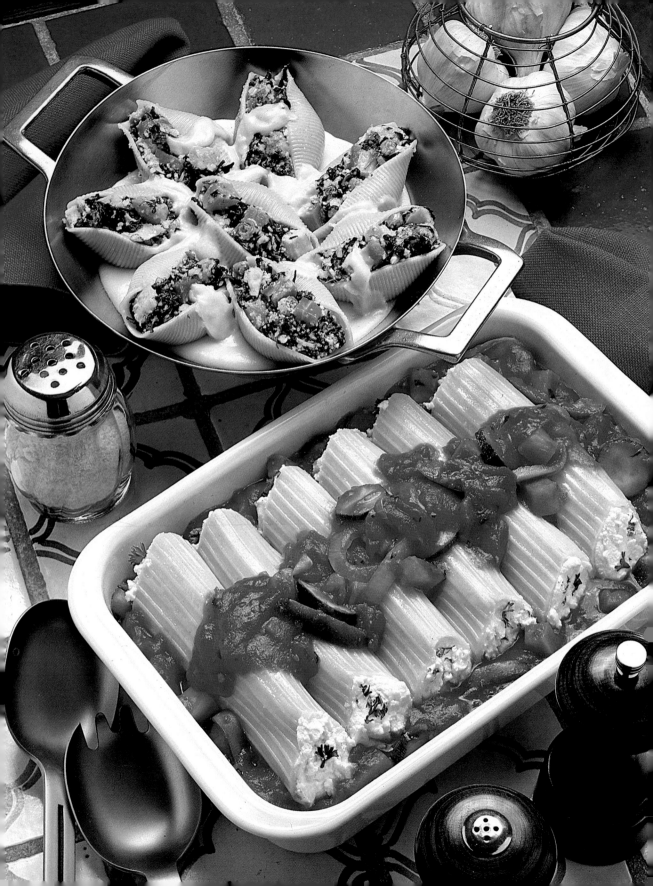

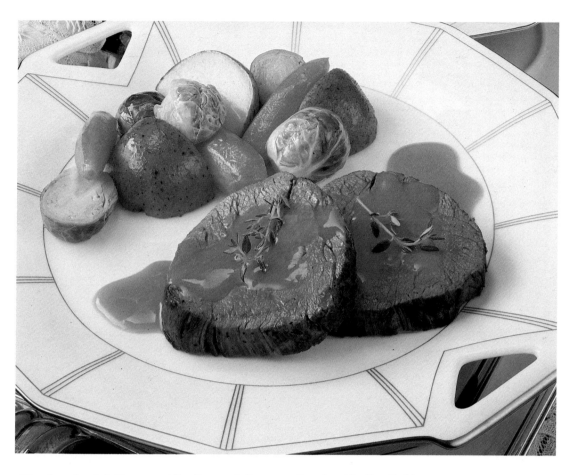

Manicotti with Ratatouille Sauce / Savory Jumbo Shells (left)

Poached Beef Tenderloin with Steamed Vegetables

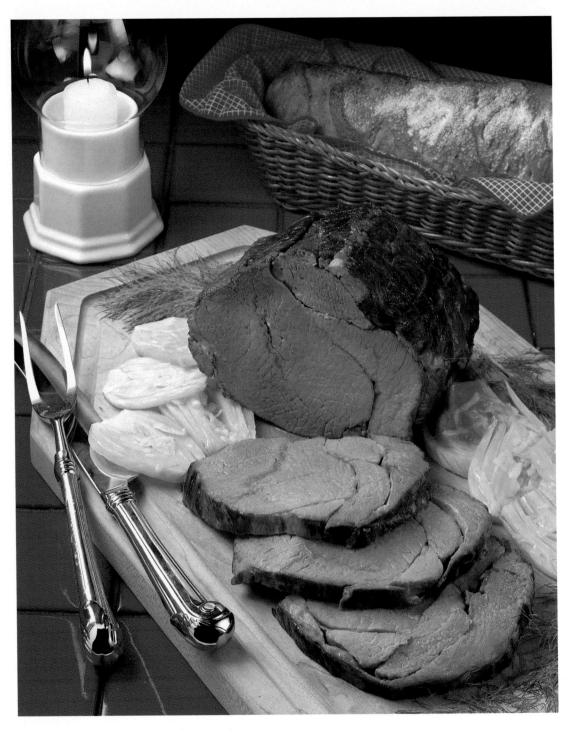

Microwave Beef Roast and Fennel Parmesan

Chicken Tarragon

8   split chicken breasts, skinned, boned (4 ounces each)
     Pepper to taste
1½ teaspoons chopped fresh tarragon
1   tablespoon white wine vinegar
⅔   cup all-purpose flour
     Pepper to taste
3   tablespoons liquid oil
18   medium mushroom caps

*M*arinate the chicken breasts in the taragon and white wine vinegar. Cover and refrigerate for 2 hours. Drain, dredge in flour, and season to taste. Brown in hot oil. Remove and place in baking dish. Sauté mushrooms in the same oil, and spoon over the chicken breasts. Cover and bake at 350° for 35 to 40 minutes.

Exchange Values
Per Serving:
½ Vegetable
½ Bread
3 Meat

218 Calories
(28% from Fat)
9.2gm Carbohydrates
28.6gm Protein
6.8gm Fat
67mg Cholesterol
77mg Sodium
450mg Potassium

Chicken Teriyaki

4   split chicken breasts, skinned (5 ounces each with bone)
2   cups water
¼   cup chopped green pepper
¼   cup chopped mushrooms
¼   cup chopped water chestnuts
¼   cup snow peas
1   15¼ ounce can unsweetened pineapple chunks

*B*oil the chicken breasts in 2 cups of water until the meat is tender and easily removed from the bone. Retain the broth. Add the chicken meat, vegetables, and pineapple, and bring to a rapid boil. Reduce the heat and simmer for 30 minutes or until the vegetables are tender. Serve over cooked seasoned rice (not included in analysis).

Exchange Values
Per Serving:
½ Vegetable
1 Fruit
3 Meat

205 Calories
(7% from Fat)
19.8gm Carbohydrates
27.6gm Protein
1.6gm Fat
67mg Cholesterol
78mg Sodium
492mg Potassium

Citrus Broiled Chicken

EIGHT SERVINGS

8 chicken breasts, split and skinned (5 ounces each with bone)

■ ■ ■

¼ cup lemon juice
¼ cup sugar-free orange jelly
¼ cup sugar-free apricot jelly
½ cup hot water
1 tablespoon dark prepared mustard
¼ teaspoon thyme leaves
¼ teaspoon crushed marjoram leaves

Exchange Values
Per Serving:
3 Meat

150 Calories
(23% from Fat)
0.7gm Carbohydrates
26.2gm Protein
3.9gm Fat
72mg Cholesterol
92mg Sodium
221mg Potassium

*P*lace the chicken pieces in a 5 quart Dutch oven. Cover with enough water to completely submerge. Bring to a boil, then reduce the heat. Cover and simmer for 10 minutes. Remove from the heat and drain off the liquid. In a small bowl, combine the remaining ingredients. Place the chicken pieces in a large, shallow non-metal container. Pour the marinade over the chicken and marinate in the refrigerator for 2 to 4 hours, basting several times. Drain the chicken, and reserve the marinade. When ready to barbecue, place the chicken bone-side down on a grill 4 to 6 inches from medium-hot coals, and brush with marinade. Cook for 20 to 30 minutes or until the chicken is tender, turning and brushing frequently with marinade.

Gingered Lime Chicken

SIX SERVINGS

½ teaspoon pepper
2 large garlic cloves, minced
1 tablespoon fresh minced ginger
1 cup all-purpose flour
6 split chicken breasts, skinned (5 ounces each with bone)
¼ cup safflower oil
   Juice of 1 lime
   Parsley
   Lime wedges

Exchange Values
Per Serving:
1 Bread
3 Meat
2 Fat

Combine pepper, garlic, and ginger with the flour. Coat the chicken well in the flour mixture. Heat the oil in a frying pan and cook the chicken pieces until lightly brown on both sides. Remove and place in a baking dish. Squeeze the lime juice over both pieces. Cover and bake at 350° for 30 minutes. Remove the cover and bake an additional 10 minutes. Remove and place on a serving dish. Garnish with parsley and lime wedges.

285 Calories
(35% from Fat)
16.3gm Carbohydrates
28.5gm Protein
11.2gm Fat
66mg Cholesterol
78mg Sodium
311mg Potassium

Herbed Chicken

SIXTEEN SERVINGS

2 **whole chickens (or 1 large turkey)**
7 **cloves garlic**
2 **bay leaves**

■ ■ ■

⅓ **cup liquid margarine**
1 **teaspoon pepper**
½ **teaspoon thyme leaves**
½ **teaspoon rubbed sage**
½ **teaspoon oregano**
½ **teaspoon marjoram**
½ **teaspoon dry basil**

Exchange Values
Per Serving:
2 Meat
1 Fat

132 Calories
(43% from Fat)
0.0gm Carbohydrates
17.4gm Protein
6.3gm Fat
48mg Cholesterol
88mg Sodium
142mg Potassium

Rinse and dry the chickens or turkey. Rub the skin with a clove of the garlic. Stuff the cavity with the bay leaves and garlic cloves. Melt the margarine in a saucepan and add the remaining ingredients. Place 1 tablespoon of margarine-herbed mixture in the cavities, and brush the remaining mixture over the skins. Bake at 350° for 1½ hours or until tender. Discard the cooked skin. Each serving is 2 ounces of cooked meat.

Roasted Orange Chicken

SIXTEEN SERVINGS

2 whole chickens
1 orange, halved
2 whole oranges

■ ■ ■

⅓ cup liquid margarine
1½ teaspoons salt substitute or "Mrs. Dash"
1 teaspoon pepper
½ teaspoon thyme leaves
½ teaspoon rubbed sage
½ teaspoon oregano
½ teaspoon marjoram
½ teaspoon dry basil

*Exchange Values
Per Serving:*
2 Meat
1 Fat

*145 Calories
(40% from Fat)*
3.4gm Carbohydrates
17.7gm Protein
6.4gm Fat
48mg Cholesterol
89mg Sodium
195mg Potassium

*R*inse and dry the chickens. Rub the skins with the orange halves. Stuff the cavities with the whole oranges. In a saucepan, melt the margarine and add the remaining ingredients. Place 1 tablespoon of margarine-herb mixture in each cavity. Place the chickens on a foil-lined pan. Baste the chickens with the remaining herb mixture. Bake at 350° for 1½ hours or until tender. Discard the cooked skin. Each serving is 2 ounces of cooked meat.

Poultry and Rice Pilaf

EIGHT SERVINGS

2 cups unsalted chicken broth
½ cup long grain rice
½ teaspoon cinnamon
¼ teaspoon black pepper
3 tablespoons pine nuts

■ ■ ■

8 split chicken breasts, skinned, boned (4 ounces each)

■ ■ ■

2 tablespoons liquid margarine
½ clove garlic, mashed
Juice of ½ lemon
1 teaspoon oregano
Parsley for garnish

*Exchange Values
Per Serving:*
½ Bread
3 Meat
1 Fat

*226 Calories
(28% from Fat)*
11.4gm Carbohydrates
28.3gm Protein
7.0gm Fat

Combine the broth, rice, cinnamon, pepper, and pine nuts. Cook for 5 minutes over low heat, stirring often. Reduce the heat and simmer for 20 minutes or until the rice is done. Place the boned chicken in a foil-lined pan. Combine the melted margarine, garlic, lemon, and oregano, and brush on the chicken. Seal the foil. Bake at 350° for 30 minutes. Uncover for the last 10 minutes. Serve the hot rice mixture on large platter topped with chicken pieces. Garnish with parsley.

66mg Cholesterol
107mg Sodium
508mg Potassium

Stir Fry Chicken

EIGHT SERVINGS

1 cup unsalted chicken broth
2 tablespoons soy sauce
2 tablespoons Worcestershire sauce
¼ teaspoon garlic powder
½ cup onion, chopped
1 cup celery, diced

2 cups cooked chicken
1 6-ounce can bean sprouts
1 6-ounce can bamboo shoots
1 8-ounce can sliced water chestnuts
1 6-ounce can sliced mushrooms
1 6-ounce package frozen snow peas

Exchange Values
Per Serving:
2 Vegetable
2 Meat

154 Calories
(26% from Fat)
9.4gm Carbohydrates
19.1gm Protein
4.5gm Fat
50mg Cholesterol
397mg Sodium
544mg Potassium

Heat the broth in a saucepan until simmering. Add the soy sauce, Worcestershire sauce, garlic powder, onion, and celery. Cook for about 5 or 6 minutes. Add the remaining ingredients except the rice, and cook for 10 minutes. Serve over hot rice (not included in analysis).

Kiwi Chicken

EIGHT SERVINGS

8 split chicken breasts, skinned (5 ounces each with bone)
½ cup all-purpose flour
   White pepper and paprika
¼ safflower oil
1 cup unsalted chicken broth
4 garlic cloves, smashed
4 kiwi fruit
   Chopped parsley

*D*redge the chicken in flour and seasonings. Sauté the chicken in hot oil until golden brown. Place in a Dutch oven. Pour chicken broth over. Crush the garlic cloves and place around the chicken. Peel and slice the kiwi and arrange around the chicken. Cover and bake at 350° for 1 hour or until the chicken is tender. Sprinkle with chopped parsley and serve from the Dutch oven.

Exchange Values
Per Serving:
1 Fruit
3 Meat
½ Fat

211 Calories
(23% from Fat)
10.6gm Carbohydrates
28.2gm Protein
5.4gm Fat
67mg Cholesterol
76mg Sodium
516mg Potassium

Vegetable and Chicken Outdoor Bake

EIGHT SERVINGS

1 pound diced, cooked chicken
1 bunch fresh broccoli
1 bunch fresh cauliflower
2 stalks celery
1 medium onion, chopped
2 carrots, diced
2 tablespoons liquid margarine

*C*ombine all of the ingredients except the margarine in a large piece of foil (dull side out). Sprinkle with melted margarine and seal all edges of the foil. Place on a hot grill and cover. Bake for 20 to 25 minutes, until heated throughout.

Exchange Values
Per Serving:
1½ Vegetable
2 Meat
1 Fat

176 Calories
(44% from Fat)
6.5gm Carbohydrates
18.3gm Protein
8.7gm Fat
50mg Cholesterol
126mg Sodium
461mg Potassium

Stuffed Chicken Breasts

TWO SERVINGS

1 whole chicken breast, split, skinned and boned
½ cup chopped Golden Delicious apples
2 tablespoons shredded low-cholesterol imitation Cheddar cheese
1 tablespoon fine dry bread crumbs
1 tablespoon liquid margarine
¼ cup dry white wine
   Water
1½ teaspoons cornstarch
   Chopped parsley

Exchange Values Per Serving:
½ Bread
3 Meat
1 Fat

266 Calories
(40% from Fat)
8.2gm Carbohydrates
30.3gm Protein
11.8gm Fat
69mg Cholesterol
228mg Sodium
335mg Potassium

*F*latten the chicken breasts between sheets of waxed paper to ¼-inch thickness. Combine the apple, cheese, and bread crumbs, and divide between the chicken breasts. Roll up each chicken breast and secure with toothpicks. Melt the margarine in a 7-inch skillet and brown the chicken in the margarine. Add the wine and ¼ cup water, cover, and simmer for 15 to 20 minutes or until the chicken is no longer pink. Remove the chicken from the pan. Combine 1 tablespoon of water with the cornstarch and stir into the juices in the pan. Cook and stir until thickened. Pour the gravy over the chicken and garnish with parsley.

Oven-Baked Chicken Livers

FOUR SERVINGS

1 pound chicken livers
½ cup skim milk
1½ cups Rice Krispies
1 cube chicken bouillon dissolved in ½ cup water
1 medium onion, slivered
   Paprika

Exchange Values Per Serving:
1 Bread
3 Meat

203 Calories
(20% from Fat)
15.5gm Carbohydrates
23.7gm Protein
4.4gm Fat
629mg Cholesterol
374mg Sodium
260mg Potassium

*S*oak the chicken livers in milk. Roll in Rice Krispies and place in a baking dish. Pour the bouillon and onion over the liver, and sprinkle with paprika. Cover and bake at 350° for 1 hour or until tender.

Zesty Chicken Italiano

EIGHT SERVINGS

2   tablespoons liquid margarine
1   pound boneless chicken breasts, cut into 1-inch pieces
1   garlic clove, minced
1½ cups thinly slized zucchini
1½ cups sliced fresh mushrooms
1   15-ounce can tomato sauce
1   14½-ounce can tomatoes, undrained and quartered
1½ teaspoons oregano
½   teaspoon lemon-pepper
⅛   teaspoon cayenne pepper (optional)
8   ounces capellini or vermicelli, uncooked
½   cup grated Parmesan cheese

Exchange Values
Per Serving:
1½ Bread
2 Meat
1 Fat
1 Vegetable

263 Calories
(20% from Fat)
32.0gm Carbohydrates
21.0gm Protein
5.9gm Fat
37mg Cholesterol
493mg Sodium
728mg Potassium

*M*elt the margarine in a large skillet. Sauté the chicken pieces until lightly browned. Add the garlic, zucchini, and mushrooms, and sauté for 2 minutes. Stir in the remaining ingredients except the pasta and Parmesan cheese, and simmer uncovered for 10 minutes to blend the flavors and thicken the sauce. Meanwhile, cook the pasta according to the package directions. Drain. Serve the hot cooked pasta with the sauce. Sprinkle with Parmesan cheese.

Turkey with Cranberry-Apple Sauce

EIGHT SERVINGS

2   frozen turkey breasts, thawed
2   teaspoons thyme leaves
    Pepper to taste
2   medium onions, quartered
2   garlic cloves

■ ■ ■

2   cups coarsely chopped red apples
1   tablespoon liquid margarine
3   cups cranberry-apple drink
¼   cup cornstarch
1   tablespoon orange rind
1   cup whole berry cranberry sauce

Exchange Values
Per Serving:
½ Vegetable
2 Fruit
2 Meat
½ Fat

270 Calories
(15% from Fat)
40.6gm Carbohydrates
17.3gm Protein
4.4gm Fat

*R*ub one teaspoon of thyme inside and outside of each turkey breast and sprinkle with pepper. Place onion and garlic inside each breast cavity. Place the breasts skin side up on the rack in a roasting pan. Bake at 350° for 2½ to 3 hours or until the internal temperature reaches 170° and the turkey is tender. Let the turkey stand for 15 minutes before slicing.

Sauté apples in margarine, and set aside. Add the cranberry-apple drink to the cornstarch in a medium saucepan, and blend well. Add the cranberry sauce and orange rinds. Cook over medium heat until the mixture boils and thickens, stirring constantly. Add the apples and stir until thoroughly heated. Serve ½ cup of the sauce with 2 ounces of sliced turkey.

43mg Cholesterol
59mg Sodium
299mg Potassium

Ale-Poached Fish with Pimiento Sauce

EIGHT SERVINGS

1½ pounds black sea bass fillets (or other), fresh or frozen
1   cup water
1   cup light beer
1   small onion, sliced
1   teaspoon Worcestershire sauce
3   peppercorns
1   clove garlic

■ ■ ■

2   tablespoons liquid margarine
2   tablespoons all-purpose flour
1   10¾-ounce can chicken broth
3   tablespoons chopped pimiento
1   teaspoon curry powder
1   teaspoon lemon juice
¾   teaspoon sugar

Exchange Values
Per Serving:
2 Meat
1 Fat

153 Calories
(37% from Fat)
4.0gm Carbohydrates
17.4gm Protein
6.3gm Fat
58mg Cholesterol
218mg Sodium
391mg Potassium

*T*haw the fish if frozen. Remove the skin and bones. Combine the water, beer, onion, Worcestershire sauce, peppercorns, and garlic in a 10-inch skillet and bring to a gentle boil. Place the fillets in the poaching liquid, cover, and simmer for 5 to 10 minutes or until the fish flakes easily when tested with a fork. Carefully remove the fish to a warm platter.

Melt the margarine in a medium saucepan. Stir in the flour. Add the chicken broth gradually and cook until thick and smooth, stirring constantly. Add the pimiento, curry powder, lemon juice, and sugar and heat through. Pour the sauce over the fish and serve.

Broiled Fish Steaks and Herbs

EIGHT SERVINGS

1	**tablespoon liquid margarine**
1	**tablespoon finely chopped parsley**
1½	**teaspoons celery salt**
½	**teaspoon crumbled oregano leaves**
¼	**teaspoon white pepper**

■ ■ ■

1½	**pounds fish steaks**
¼	**cup white wine**
1	**tablespoon lemon juice**

■ ■ ■

Fresh parsley for garnish

Exchange Values
Per Serving:
2 Meat

84 Calories
(21% from Fat)
0.3gm Carbohydrates
15.2gm Protein
2.0gm Fat
37mg Cholesterol
452mg Sodium
360mg Potassium

*M*elt the margarine in a small saucepan and add next four ingredients. Arrange the fish in baking dish and brush the herb butter over the fish. Add the white wine and lemon juice over the fish. Cover and bake at 350° for 30 minutes. Uncover and bake 5 more minutes. The fish should flake easily with a fork when done. Garnish with parsley.

Cornflake-Breaded Baked Fish

SIX SERVINGS

1	**pound fresh or frozen fish fillets (sole, flounder, or perch)**
	Juice of 1 lemon
¼	**teaspoon salt substitute**
	Dash fresh ground pepper
2	**tablespoons safflower oil**
⅓	**cup cornflake crumbs**

Exchange Values
Per Serving:
2 Meat
1 Fat

130 Calories
(38% from Fat)
4.9gm Carbohydrates
14.7gm Protein
5.5gm Fat
36mg Cholesterol
120mg Sodium
290mg Potassium

*W*ash and dry the fish fillets, and cut into serving size pieces, allowing for shrinkage. Rub each piece with the lemon juice. Season and then dip in oil. Drain. Coat the outside of each piece with cornflakes. Arrange in a single layer in a baking dish that has been sprayed beforehand. Bake at 350° for 30 minutes or until the fish flakes.

Fish Almondine

½   cup slivered almonds
1½ pounds bluefish, boned and cleaned
1   tablespoon liquid margarine
½   teaspoon parsley
     Paprika, pepper
     Lemon wedges

Exchange Values
Per Serving:
3 Meat
2 Fat

203 Calories
(47% from Fat)
3.2gm Carbohydrates
23.4gm Protein
10.9gm Fat
49mg Cholesterol
81mg Sodium
587mg Potassium

*A*rrange the almonds in a single layer on a cookie sheet and bake at 350° for 4 to 5 minutes or until golden brown. Place the fish in an ungreased baking pan. Arrange the toasted almonds on the top of the fish. Drizzle melted margarine over the fish and almonds. Sprinkle with parsley, paprika and pepper to taste. Bake at 350° for 20 to 25 minutes, or until the fish flakes easily. Serve with a lemon wedge on top of each piece.

Flounder Bake

8   ounces flounder fillets
4   ounces evaporated skim milk
    Paprika, pepper, and salt substitute to taste
½   tablespoon lemon juice
¼   cup chopped onion
4   ounces sliced mushrooms
2   stalks celery, chopped
1   cup chopped cauliflower
1   cup chopped broccoli
1   cup slivered carrots
2   tablespoons margarine, melted

Exchange Values
Per Serving:
2 Vegetable
2 Meat
1 Fat

194 Calories
(42% from Fat)
11.8gm Carbohydrates
18.0gm Protein
8.9gm Fat
37mg Cholesterol
226mg Sodium
808mg Potassium

*M*arinate the fish fillets in milk for 15 minutes. Drain. Sprinkle the fillets with paprika, pepper, salt substitute, and lemon juice. Place in a foil tent inside a baking dish. Cover with the vegetables and drizzle with margarine. Bake at 350° for 15 to 20 minutes or until tender.

Hot Tuna and Potato Bake

EIGHT SERVINGS

3 7-ounce cans water-packed tuna, drained
1 3-ounce can sliced mushrooms
1 tablespoon Worcestershire sauce
½ teaspoon Tabasco sauce

   ■ ■ ■

2 tablespoons vinegar
3 cups potatoes, cooked and diced

   ■ ■ ■

¼ cup liquid margarine
¼ cup thinly sliced onion
¼ cup thinly sliced celery
¼ cup all-purpose flour
1 teaspoon dry mustard
2 cups skim milk
1 cup plain lowfat yogurt

Exchange Values
Per Serving:
½ Milk
1 Bread
3 Meat
1 Fat

246 Calories
(24% from Fat)
20.9gm Carbohydrates
24.4gm Protein
6.8gm Fat
63mg Cholesterol
404mg Sodium
629mg Potassium

*C*ombine the tuna, mushrooms, Worcestershire sauce, and Tabasco sauce. In a separate bowl, combine the vinegar and potatoes. Melt the margarine in a sauté pan and simmer the onion and celery until tender. Add the flour and dry mustard, and remove from the heat. Gradually add the milk and yogurt, and stir until combined. Place ½ of the potatoes in a large casserole dish. Top with half of the tuna mixture and half of the sauce mixture. Repeat the layers. Bake at 350° for 35 minutes.

Tuna and Noodle Casserole Bake

SIX SERVINGS

1½ cups dry wide noodles, 1-inch pieces
6 cups water
¾ teaspoon salt substitute

   ■ ■ ■

¼ cup finely chopped celery
¼ cup finely chopped onion

Exchange Values
Per Serving:
1 Vegetable
2 Bread
3 Meat

4   teaspoons liquid margarine
    Dash white pepper
2   cups canned tomatoes, crushed
2   7-ounce cans water packed tuna, drained
4   tablespoons Parmesan cheese

341 Calories
(12% from Fat)
46.8gm Carbohydrates
26.2gm Protein
4.7gm Fat
63mg Cholesterol
425mg Sodium
744mg Potassium

*C*ook the noodles in 6 cups of salted water. Drain and rinse in cold water. Sauté the celery and onion in margarine. When the vegetables are tender, add the pepper, tomatoes, and tuna. Add the sautéed mixture to the noodles and place in a sprayed baking dish. Sprinkle the top with Parmesan cheese. Bake at 350° for 30 minutes.

Tuna Potato Casserole

SIX SERVINGS

1½ cups cooked enriched noodles
1   7-ounce can tuna, drained
4   ounces peas
½   cup canned mushrooms, drained
4   ounces evaporated skim milk
2   tablespoons onion flakes
    Dash pepper
1   tablespoon Worcestershire sauce
½   teaspoon Tabasco sauce
1   cup cubed potatoes
¼   cup copped celery
¼   cup crushed Ritz crackers

Exchange Values
Per Serving:
1½ Bread
1 Meat

161 Calories
(8% from Fat)
22.8gm Carbohydrates
13.4gm Protein
1.5gm Fat
36mg Cholesterol
270mg Sodium
427mg Potassium

*C*ombine all of the ingredients except the cracker crumbs and place in a casserole dish. Sprinkle the top with the crumbs. Bake covered at 350° for 30 to 40 minutes, until the potatoes are tender. Uncover for the last 10 minutes of cooking time to brown the top.

Trout Bake

4 5-ounce trout fillets, halved
1 cup skim milk
1 cup Rice Krispies
3 tablespoons liquid margarine
½ cup roasted almonds

Soak the trout in the milk for 1 hour before cooking. Drain. In a separate bowl, combine the Rice Krispies and melted margarine. Dredge the trout in Rice Krispies and place in a baking dish. Sprinkle the tops of the fillets with almonds. Bake uncovered at 350° for 30 minutes or until the fish flakes well.

Exchange Values
Per Serving:
2 Meat
2 Fat

191 Calories
(53% from Fat)
5.2gm Carbohydrates
16.9gm Protein
11.3gm Fat
41mg Cholesterol
108mg Sodium
436mg Potassium

Crab Imperial

1 pound cooked crab meat
½ cup chopped pimiento
½ cup finely chopped celery
2 slices crustless low-calorie bread (40 calories/slice)
2 egg whites (or egg substitute) beaten
1 cup plain lowfat yogurt
   Dash Worcestershire sauce
⅛ teaspoon cayenne pepper
1 teaspoon dry mustard
¼ teaspoon salt substitute
   Juice of ½ lemon
   Paprika

Exchange Values
Per Serving:
2 Meat

96 Calories
(16% from Fat)
5.9gm Carbohydrates
13.9gm Protein
1.7gm Fat
32mg Cholesterol
667mg Sodium
332mg Potassium

Combine the crab meat, pimiento, and celery in a mixing bowl. Crumble the slices of bread and add to the mixture. Gently add the egg white, yogurt, Worcestershire, cayenne, mustard, salt substitute, and lemon juice. Place in a sprayed casserole dish. Top with a sprinkle of paprika. Bake at 400° for 15 to 20 minutes, until lightly brown.

Lettuce-Baked Lobster Tails

SIX SERVINGS

6 **lobster tails (½ pound each)**
½ **cup liquid margarine**
¼ **to ½ teaspoon garlic powder**
   Paprika
   10 to 12 lettuce leaves, rinsed and drained

*T*haw the lobster if frozen. Fan cut the tails by cutting off the under shell, leaving the tail fan and upper shell in place. Place the lobster shell-side down on a baking sheet. Combine the margarine with the garlic powder and brush onto the lobster meat. Sprinkle with paprika. Cover the tails completely with damp lettuce leaves and bake at 400° for 15 to 20 minutes or until the lobster meat is opaque white and tender. Discard the lettuce leaves.

*Exchange Values
Per Serving:*
4 Meat
2 Fat

279 Calories
(54% from Fat)
0.9gm Carbohydrates
30.1gm Protein
16.7gm Fat
150mg Cholesterol
149mg Sodium
20mg Potassium

Seaman's Fish Bake

SIX SERVINGS

½ **cup enriched cornmeal**
¼ **teaspoon nutmeg**
½ **teaspoon paprika**
¼ **teaspoon pepper**
1 **pound fresh or frozen cod, halibut or sole fillets, thawed**
¼ **cup egg substitute**
2 **tablespoons skim milk**
2 **tablespoons margarine, melted**

*C*ombine the cornmeal, nutmeg, paprika, and pepper. Dredge the fish in the egg and milk mixture. Coat with the cornmeal mixture and place in a shallow pan. Drizzle with melted margarine. Bake for 15 to 20 minutes or until golden brown.

*Exchange Values
Per Serving:*
½ Bread
2 Meat
1 Fat

146 Calories
(30% from Fat)
8.5gm Carbohydrates
15.9gm Protein
4.9gm Fat
33mg Cholesterol
99mg Sodium
379mg Potassium

Baked Spicy Shrimp

SIX SERVINGS

1 teaspoon salt substitute
1½ pounds shrimp, shelled and deveined
2 tablespoons safflower oil
1 garlic clove, minced
¼ cup chopped green onions
¼ cup chopped green pepper
½ cup dry white wine
8 drops Tabasco sauce
¼ teaspoon ground mustard
   Juice of 1 lemon
½ cup soft bread crumbs

*Exchange Values
Per Serving:*
2 Meat
1 Fat
½ Bread

*163 Calories
(35% from Fat)*
9.1gm Carbohydrates
16.7gm Protein
6.3gm Fat
115mg Cholesterol
176mg Sodium
440mg Potassium

Sprinkle the salt substitute over the shrimp on all sides. Heat the oil in 12-inch skillet over moderate heat. Add the garlic, shrimp, onion and green pepper, and sauté for 2 or 3 minutes. Reduce the heat and stir in the wine, seasonings, and lemon juice. Cover and simmer for 5 minutes. Place the shrimp in a single layer in a sprayed quart baking dish. Pour the sauce evenly over the tops of the shrimp and top with crumbs. Bake at 350° for 15 minutes or until tender.

Rock Shrimp and Oyster Manquechou

SIX SERVINGS

4 slices bacon
1 large onion, finely chopped
1 teaspoon finely chopped garlic
½ cup chopped green pepper
2 cups fresh or defrosted frozen corn
2½ cups canned peeled tomatoes, chopped and drained
   (reserve liquid)
½ pound peeled and deveined rock shrimp, thawed if frozen
½ pint oysters, drained (reserve liquid)
   Water added to oyster liquid to make 1 cup
¼ teaspoon cayenne pepper

*Exchange Values
Per Serving:*
1 Vegetable
1 Bread
2 Meat
½ Fat

*165 Calories
(18% from Fat)*
18.6gm Carbohydrates
16.9gm Protein
3.5gm Fat

*F*ry the bacon until crisp in a heavy 4-quart casserole. Drain the fat. Add the onion, garlic, and green pepper, and cook until the onion is translucent but not brown. Stir in the corn and tomatoes. Add the tomato liquid, reserved oyster liquid, and cayenne pepper. Simmer for 10 minutes or until the corn is tender. Add the shrimp and oysters and cook for 2 minutes or until the edges of the oysters begin to curl. Serve at once.

80.3mg Cholesterol
440mg Sodium
462mg Potassium

Shrimp and Mushrooms

SIX SERVINGS

1	tablespoon margarine
1½	cups cooked shrimp, drained and rinsed
½	cup chopped celery
2	tablespoons minced onion
1	8-ounce can sliced mushrooms, drained

■ ■ ■

½	cup beef bouillon
½	cup water, divided
1	tablespoon cornstarch
¼	teaspoon nutmeg
	Dash pepper
1	teaspoon soy sauce

■ ■ ■

2	cups hot cooked rice

Exchange Values Per Serving:
1 Vegetable
1 Bread
2 Meat

170 Calories
(14% from Fat)
19.7gm Carbohydrates
15.4gm Protein
2.7gm Fat
128mg Cholesterol
681mg Sodium
255mg Potassium

*M*elt the margarine in a large skillet. Add the shrimp and cook for 4 to 6 minutes, stirring often. Add the celery, onion, and mushrooms. Cook, stirring over high heat, for about 1½ to 2 minutes.

Dissolve the bouillon cube in ¼ cup of boiling water. Combine the cornstarch and ¼ cup of cold water. Add the nutmeg, pepper, soy sauce, and bouillon broth, and pour over the shrimp mixture, cooking and stirring until thick and clear. Spoon the shrimp over the rice.

Leek and Mussel Poach

TWELVE SERVINGS

½ cup julienne-cut celery
½ cup julienne-cut carrots
½ cup julienne-cut zucchini

   ■ ■ ■

1 cup water (reserved from cooking vegetables)
1 cup dry white wine
½ cup leeks or scallions, finely sliced
4 dozen mussels

   ■ ■ ■

2 pounds haddock or cod

   ■ ■ ■

½ cup skim milk
¼ cup all-purpose flour
¼ teaspoon nutmeg
  Pepper to taste
  Paprika to taste
¼ cup liquid margarine

   ■ ■ ■

2 tablespoons chopped fresh parsley

Exchange Values
Per Serving:
½ Bread
2 Meat
1 Fat

155 Calories
(31% from Fat)
6.2gm Carbohydrates
19.7gm Protein
5.4gm Fat
54mg Cholesterol
211mg Sodium
457mg Potassium

*C*ook the julienne vegetables in a large saucepan in water to cover until tender but still firm. Drain and reserve 1 cup of water. Set the vegetables aside. Bring the water, wine and chopped leeks to a simmer. Scrub and debeard the mussels, and add to the leeks. Cover and steam. Continue to steam for 5 minutes after the mussels have opened. Remove about half from their shells and reserve the rest, keeping warm for garnish.

Strain the liquid from the steaming mussels into a large skillet and add the fish. Cover and gently simmer for 8 to 10 minutes, until the fish flakes easily. Transfer to an ovenproof platter and keep warm. Reduce the liquid quickly to ½ cup. Add the skim milk, flour, seasonings, and margarine in small pieces, whisking constantly. Add the shelled mussels and parsley, and heat through. Pour the sauce over the fish, top with the julienne of vegetables, and garnish with the remaining mussels.

Baked Beef Tenderloin with Vegetables

SIXTEEN SERVINGS

1   4-pound beef tenderloin roast
¼ cup soy sauce
2   tablespoons Worcestershire sauce
    Garlic to taste

    ■ ■ ■

2   onions, quartered
1   pound fresh mushrooms, sliced
4   to 6 ribs celery, sliced diagonally
6   carrots, cleaned and diced
1   lemon, sliced thin
¼ cup water

Exchange Values
Per Serving:
1 Vegetable
3 Meat

203 Calories
(36% from Fat)
6.4gm Carbohydrates
25.4gm Protein
8.1gm Fat
71mg Cholesterol
301mg Sodium
631mg Potassium

*M*arinate the tenderloin overnight in the combined soy sauce, Worcestershire sauce, and garlic. Before cooking, add the remaining ingredients to the pan. Cover and bake at 350° for 1½ hours.

Beef and Noodles

SIX SERVINGS

1   pound beef, cut into 2 x 2½-inch strips (or lean ground beef)
½ cup sliced onion
1   garlic clove, minced
2   tablespoons oil
1   6-ounce can mushrooms, drained
2   drops Tabasco sauce
1   tablespoon Worcestershire sauce
1   tablespoon soy sauce
¼ teaspoon pepper
¼ teaspoon paprika
    Dash nutmeg
1   10¾-ounce can condensed tomato soup

    ■ ■ ■

    Cooked noodles

Exchange Values
Per Serving:
½ Bread
2 Meat
1 Fat

289 Calories
(65% from Fat)
9.4gm Carbohydrates
15.1gm Protein
21.0gm Fat
57mg Cholesterol
682mg Sodium
412mg Potassium

*S*auté the beef, onion and garlic in oil. When browned, add the mushrooms, seasonings, and soup. Simmer until the beef is tender. Serve over the cooked noodles (not included in analysis).

Holiday Beef Steaks
with Vegetable Sauté and Hot Mustard Sauce

SIX SERVINGS

1 pound boneless beef top loin steaks, cut 1-inch thick
½ cup plain lowfat yogurt
1 teaspoon cornstarch
¼ cup condensed beef broth
2 teaspoons coarse-grained mustard
1 teaspoon *each* prepared grated horseradish and Dijon-style mustard
½ teaspoon lemon-pepper
1 16-ounce package frozen whole green beans
1 cup quartered large mushrooms
1 tablespoon liquid margarine
¼ cup water

Exchange Values
Per Serving:
1 Vegetable
2 Meat
1 Fat

206 Calories
(49% from Fat)
8.9gm Carbohydrates
17.8gm Protein
11.3gm Fat
43mg Cholesterol
160mg Sodium
258mg Potassium

*P*lace the yogurt and cornstarch in a medium saucepan and stir until blended. Stir in the beef broth, coarse-grained mustard, horseradish, and Dijon-style mustard. Set aside.

Press an equal amount of lemon-pepper into the surface of the steaks. Place the steaks on a rack in a broiler pan and place the steaks 3 to 4 inches from the heat in the oven. Broil the steaks about 15 minutes for rare, 20 minutes for medium, turning once.

Meanwhile cook the beans and mushrooms in margarine in a large frying pan over medium heat for 6 minutes, stirring occasionally, until the beans are tender. Cook the reserved sauce over medium-low heat for 5 minutes, stirring until the sauce is slightly thickened. Serve the steaks and vegetables with the sauce.

Fall Apple Pot Roast

TWELVE SERVINGS

3 to 4 pounds beef blade pot roast
2 tablespoons oil
¼ cup all-purpose flour
¼ teaspoon pepper
2 medium onions, sliced
½ cup water

Exchange Values
Per Serving:
½ Vegetable
½ Fruit
3 Meat
½ Fat

1 acorn squash or piece large winter squash (about 1 pound)
2 tart apples, cored and quartered

*T*rim the surface fat from the roast and fry it in oil in a large skillet. Mix the flour and pepper together and rub the mixture all over the meat. Brown the meat in the fat, turning to brown on all sides. Pour off the excess drippings. Add the onions and cook until they are tender but not browned. Add the water. Cover and simmer for 2 hours. Peel the squash and scrape off any seeds and stringy pulp. Slice or cube the squash and add it to the pot roast along with the apples. Cover and simmer for 30 minutes longer or until the meat and vegetables are tender.

240 Calories
(40% from Fat)
11.0gm Carbohydrates
24.4gm Protein
10.7gm Fat
69mg Cholesterol
90mg Sodium
569mg Potassium

Chinese Green Pepper Steak

SIX SERVINGS

½ cup dry sherry
4 tablespoons soy sauce
1½ pounds top sirloin beef, cut into ⅙-inch slices

■ ■ ■

1 tablespoon oil
½ teaspoon pepper
1 teaspoon shredded ginger
1 clove garlic, crushed

■ ■ ■

2 pounds fresh green peppers, each cut diagonally into pieces

■ ■ ■

1½ cups chicken broth

■ ■ ■

2 tablespoons cornstarch
¼ cup cold water
2 tablespoons soy sauce

■ ■ ■

4 cups cooked rice

Exchange Values
Per Serving:
2 Vegetable
2 Bread
3 Meat
½ Fat

433 Calories
(22% from Fat)
45.9gm Carbohydrates
31.9gm Protein
10.6gm Fat
76mg Cholesterol
1615mg Sodium
781mg Potassium

*C*ombine the sherry and 4 tablespoons of soy sauce. Marinate the beef for at least 2 hours in the mixture.

Place the oil, pepper, ginger, and garlic in a heated wok. Stir to combine. Add the beef and stir fry for 3 minutes. Add the green pepper and mix well. Add the chicken broth. Stir to combine, cover, and cook for 6 minutes.

Combine the cornstarch, water, and soy sauce. Add to the cooked beef mixture and stir continuously until the juice thickens smoothly. Serve immediately on individual plates with steamed rice.

Italian Fest

2 pounds extra lean ground beef
1 cup minced onion

■ ■ ■

3 cups water
1 garlic clove, minced
2 13-ounce cans tomato puree
1 6-ounce can tomato paste
1 teaspoon soy sauce
1 teaspoon Worcestershire sauce
2 teaspoons Italian seasoning
1 teaspoon chili powder

■ ■ ■

4 cups cooked spaghetti noodles

Exchange Values
Per Serving:
2 Vegetable
1½ Bread
3 Meat

377 Calories
(35% from Fat)
35.8gm Carbohydrates
28.6gm Protein
14.5gm Fat
70mg Cholesterol
469gm Sodium
896mg Potassium

*B*rown the ground beef and onions in a large pot. Drain the fat. Add the water, and the remaining ingredients. Stir to combine, and simmer for 30 minutes. Serve over cooked spaghetti noodles.

Lasagna Casserole

1 pound lean ground beef
½ cup chopped onion
1 6-ounce can tomato paste
1 2-pound can tomatoes, pureed in food processor
½ cup thinly sliced celery
2 teaspoons Mrs. Dash seasoning
½ teaspoon Italian seasoning
1 tablespoon Worcestershire sauce

■ ■ ■

1 pound Ricotta cheese
1 cup lowfat cottage cheese
1 8-ounce package lasagna noodles, cooked

■ ■ ■

½ pound Parmesan cheese

Exchange Values
Per Serving:
1½ Vegetable
1 Bread
3 Meat
1 Fat

358 Calories
(44% from Fat)
24.8gm Carbohydrates
25.3gm Protein
17.4gm Fat
57mg Cholesterol
652mg Sodium
564mg Potassium

*I*n a large skillet combine the ground beef, chopped onion, tomato paste, tomatoes, celery, and seasonings, and cook until the meat is brown, about 1 hour.

Puree together the Ricotta and cottage cheese in a food processor. Spray a large baking pan with cholesterol-free coating. Alternate layers of noodles, sauce, ricotta cheese, and Parmesan, repeating layers if possible. Top with Parmesan. Bake at 350° for about 30 minutes, until warmed throughout.

Old-Fashioned Beef, Macaroni and Tomato Casserole

FOUR SERVINGS

3 cups water
⅔ cup uncooked macaroni

■ ■ ■

1 pound lean ground beef
¼ cup finely chopped onions
1 tablespoon finely chopped celery
¼ cup finely chopped green pepper
1 tablespoon Worcestershire sauce
1 tablespoon soy sauce

■ ■ ■

1 cup crushed canned tomatoes
1 cup unsalted tomato juice
⅛ teaspoon pepper
¼ teaspoon basil leaves
1 teaspoon parsley flakes

Exchange Values
Per Serving:
1 Vegetable
1 Bread
3 Meat
2 Fat

412 Calories
(52% from Fat)
23.9gm Carbohydrates
24.2gm Protein
23.9gm Fat
85mg Cholesterol
643mg Sodium
773mg Potassium

*C*ook the macaroni in water until tender. Drain and rinse with cold water. Set aside. Combine the ground beef, onions, celery, green pepper, Worcestershire and soy sauces in a frying pan. Cook until the beef is browned and the vegetables are tender. Combine the canned tomatoes, tomato juice, pepper, basil leaves and parsley flakes in a large pan. Add the ground beef mixture to the tomato sauce and bring to a boil. Reduce to a simmer and stir in the macaroni. Simmer until warmed throughout.

Our Beef Oriental

TWELVE SERVINGS

2	pounds lean round steak
¼	teaspoon minced onion
¼	teaspoon minced garlic
1	tablespoon soy sauce
¼	cup water
⅛	teaspoon coarsely ground black pepper

■ ■ ■

1	beef bouillon cube
1½	cups hot water
1	16-ounce package frozen broccoli
1	16-ounce package frozen cauliflower
½	cup raw carrot strips
2½	cups sliced, fresh mushrooms
½	cup drained, sliced water chestnuts
½	cup celery

■ ■ ■

8	cups cooked and drained rice

*Exchange Values
Per Serving:*
1 Vegetable
2 Bread
2 Meat

289 Calories
(16% from Fat)
39.0gm Carbohydrates
21.2gm Protein
5.0gm Fat
46mg Cholesterol
642mg Sodium
523mg Potassiuim

*P*lace the round steak in a baking pan. Sprinkle with minced onion, minced garlic, soy sauce, water, and pepper. Bake at 350° for 30 minutes. Cut into bite-sized pieces.

Dissolve the bouillon cube in the hot water in a large pot. Add the frozen broccoli, cauliflower, carrots, mushrooms, water chestnuts, and celery. Bring to a boil and then simmer for 15 minutes. Add the cubed steak to the vegetables, and simmer an additional 15 minutes. Serve over ⅔ cup of rice.

Microwave Beef Roast and Fennel Parmesan

TWELVE SERVINGS

3	pound boneless beef chuck cross rib roast
3	large bulbs fennel (2 pounds)
½	cup water
1	clove garlic, halved
¼	cup shredded Parmesan cheese

*Exchange Values
Per Serving:*
3 Meat
1 Fat
1 Vegetable

*P*lace the roast fat-side down on a rack in a microwave-safe dish. Cover with waxed paper and microwave at medium-low or 30 percent power. Allow 18 to 20 minutes per pound. Rotate the dish ¼ turn every 20 minutes, and invert the roast at midpoint of cooking period. Edges that appear to be overcooked may be shielded with small pieces of foil during cooking. Remove the roast when a meat thermometer inserted into the thickest part registers 5° less than the doneness desired (rare to medium, 140° to 160°). Tent the roast with foil and allow to stand for 15 to 20 minutes.

Meanwhile remove the stalks and outer leaves from the fennel. Cut the bulbs lengthwise into ¼-inch thick slices, keeping the core to retain the fan shape. Place the fennel, water, and garlic in a microwave-safe casserole. Cover and cook on high for 8 minutes, rotating the dish ¼ turn after 4 minutes. Remove the garlic and pour off the water. Sprinkle the cheese over the fennel and continue cooking on high for 1 minute. Serve the fennel with the roast.

223 Calories
(44% from Fat)
5.2gm Carbohydrates
26.0gm Protein
11.0gm Fat
68mg Cholesterol
105mg Sodium
801mg Potassium

Poached Beef Tenderloin

EIGHT SERVINGS

2 **pounds beef tenderloin roast**
1 **tablespoon oil**
4 **cups water**
1 **10¾-ounce can beef broth**
1 **cup dry red wine**
2 **cloves garlic, minced**
1 **teaspoon diced marjoram leaves**
4 **black peppercorns**
3 **whole cloves**

Exchange Values
Per Serving:
3 Meat
1 Fat

246 Calories
(50% from Fat)
0gm Carbohydrates
24.0gm Protein
13.6gm Fat
73mg Cholesterol
190mg Sodium
384mg Potassium

*T*ie the beef roast with heavy string at 2 inch intervals. Brown the beef roast in oil over medium-high heat until all sides are browned. Pour off the drippings. Add the water, beef broth, wine, garlic, marjoram, peppercorns, and cloves. Bring to a boil, reduce the heat to medium-low, cover, and simmer for 10 minutes per pound. The temperature will register 130°. Do not overcook. Remove the roast to a serving platter. Cover tightly with plastic wrap or aluminum foil and allow the roast to stand for 10 minutes before carving. The roast temperature will rise approximately 10° in temperature to 140° for rare.

Remove the string and carve the roast into thin slices. Serve with Steamed Vegetables (see page 184).

Pepper Steak

FOUR SERVINGS

1 **pound flank steak**
2 **beef bouillon cubes**
½ **cup water**
1 **small onion, sliced**
1 **4-ounce can mushrooms, drained**
1 **medium green pepper, cut into thin strips**
1 **tablespoon Worcestershire sauce**
1 **tablespoon soy sauce**
  Pepper to taste

Exchange Values Per Serving:
½ Vegetable
3 Meat
1 Fat

246 Calories
(53% from Fat)
4.6gm Carbohydrates
23.1gm Protein
14.5gm Fat
59mg Cholesterol
802mg Sodium
582mg Potassium

*H*ave the flank steak cut very thin by the butcher. Place the steak strips in a baking pan and cover with water and dissolved bouillon. Layer the onions, mushrooms, and peppers over the steak. Sprinkle with Worcestershire and soy sauces. Cover and bake at 350° for 20 minutes or until the vegetables and steak are tender.

Round Steak in Wine Sauce

TEN SERVINGS

3 **pounds round steak, about 1½ inches thick**
1 **teaspoon Worcestershire sauce**
1 **teaspoon soy sauce**

■ ■ ■

2 **tablespoons liquid margarine**
1½ **cups chopped onion**
2 **tablespoons brown mustard**
1 **cup sliced fresh mushrooms**
¼ **cup dry white wine**

Exchange Values Per Serving:
½ Vegetable
3 Meat

203 Calories
(41% from Fat)
2.7gm Carbohydrates
24.9gm Protein
9.3gm Fat
70mg Cholesterol
150mg Sodium
435mg Potassium

*F*our hours before cooking, marinate the steak in the Worcestershire and soy sauces. Sauté the steak in the margarine in a large skillet. Add the remaining ingredients. Cover and simmer for 2 hours, adding 1 part wine and 1 part water to the meat as it cooks, if it becomes too dry. The meat should be tender when done.

Swedish Meatballs

1 **pound lean ground beef**
¾ **cup bread crumbs**
1 **onion, diced**
¼ **cup egg substitute**
1 **teaspoon Worcestershire sauce**
1 **tablespoon parsley flakes**
1 **teaspoon pepper**
1 **10¾-ounce can condensed cream of celery soup**
1 **soup can skim milk**

Exchange Values
Per Serving:
1 Bread
2 Meat
1 Fat

274 Calories
(45% from Fat)
17.4gm Carbohydrates
19.2gm Protein
13.7gm Fat
51mg Cholesterol
563mg Sodium
366mg Potassium

*C*ombine the ground beef, bread crumbs, onion, egg substitute, Worcestershire sauce and seasonings. Add ¼ cup of the soup to the mixture. Form into meatballs and place on a shallow baking sheet. Bake at 350° until browned. Combine the remaining soup and the milk in a saucepan. Add the meatballs and heat through, about 15 minutes.

Swiss Steak

1 **2-pound round steak**
½ **teaspoon pepper**
1 **teaspoon minced garlic**
1 **16-ounce can tomatoes, cut up, with liquid**
1 **small onion, minced**
1 **cup diced carrots**
1 **cup mushroom crowns**
½ **cup cold water**

Exchange Values
Per Serving:
1 Vegetable
3 Meat
1 Fat

298 Calories
(60% from Fat)
5.3gm Carbohydrates
23.0gm Protein
20.1gm Fat
75mg Cholesterol
160mg Sodium
566mg Potassium

*P*lace the round steak in a baking pan. Sprinkle with pepper, garlic, and onion. Combine the tomatoes, onion, carrots, mushrooms, and water, and pour over the steak. Cover and bake at 350° for 30 minutes. Uncover and continue to cook for 10 minutes more. Test for doneness.

Mostaccioli al Forno

EIGHT SERVINGS

1 10-ounce package frozen chopped spinach
2 cups Ricotta cheese
6 egg whites, lightly beaten
⅔ cup grated Parmesan cheese
1 cup shredded part skim Mozzarella cheese
⅓ cup chopped fresh parsley
¼ teaspoon pepper
8 ounces mostaccioli, uncooked
1 32-ounce jar spaghetti sauce
2 tablespoons grated Parmesan cheese

Exchange Values
Per Serving:
1 Vegetable
2 Bread
3 Meat

368 Calories
(35% from Fat)
34.7gm Carbohydrates
25.9gm Protein
14.2gm Fat
42mg Cholesterol
855mg Sodium
667mg Potassium

*C*ook the spinach according to package directions for 1 minute. Drain and press out the excess moisture. Combine the spinach, Ricotta, eggs, ⅔ cup Parmesan, ⅔ cup Mozzarella, parsley, and pepper. Set aside. Cook the mostaccioli according to the package directions for 10 minutes. Drain and combine the mostaccioli with 2½ cups of sauce. Arrange half of the mostaccioli in the bottom of an 11x7x2-inch pan or 9-inch square baking dish. Layer the spinach evenly over the mostaccioli, and cover with the remaining mostaccioli. Spread the remaining sauce over the top, and sprinkle with the remaining Mozzarella and Parmesan cheeses. Bake at 350° for 35 to 40 minutes.

Parmesan Linguine with Garlic

TEN SERVINGS

4 teaspoons olive oil
1 cup chopped zucchini
⅓ cup chopped onion
2 garlic cloves, minced
¼ pound fresh mushrooms, sliced
½ teaspoon salt substitute
   Dash crushed red pepper flakes
8 ounces linguine, prepared as directed omitting salt
2 tablespoons Parmesan cheese

Exchange Values
Per Serving:
½ Vegetable
1 Bread
½ Fat

112 Calories
(20% from Fat)
18.6gm Carbohydrates
3.7gm Protein

*H*eat the oil in a skillet. Add the zucchini, onion, and garlic, and sauté for approximately 4 minutes. Add the mushrooms, salt substitute, and red pepper flakes. Cook and stir for another 3 minutes. In a large bowl add the cooked vegetables to the linguine and toss. Sprinkle with Parmesan.

2.5gm Fat
1mg Cholesterol
20.2mg Sodium
131mg Potassium

Savory Jumbo Shells

EIGHT SERVINGS

12 to 14 jumbo pasta shells, uncooked
3 tablespoons sliced green onions
2 tablespoons liquid margarine
1 10-ounce package frozen chopped spinach,
   thawed and well drained
1 cup diced cooked chicken
1 cup diced cooked turkey
½ cup grated Parmesan cheese
4 egg whites, beaten
¾ teaspoon Italian seasoning
¼ teaspoon pepper

3 tablespoons liquid margarine
1 clove garlic, minced
3 tablespoons all-purpose flour
1½ teaspoons low-sodium instant chicken bouillon
⅛ teaspoon pepper
2 cups skim milk
½ cup grated Parmesan cheese

Exchange Values
Per Serving:
2 Bread
3 Meat
1 Fat

369 Calories
(35% from Fat)
29.0gm Carbohydrates
29.6gm Protein
14.5gm Fat
56mg Cholesterol
384mg Sodium
595mg Potassium

*C*ook the shells according to the package directions. Meanwhile combine the onions, margarine, spinach, chicken, ½ cup Parmesan cheese, egg whites, Italian seasoning, and ¼ teaspoon pepper in a mixing bowl. Fill each shell with about 3 tablespoons of filling. To prepare the cheese sauce, melt 3 tablespoons of margarine in a saucepan. Add the garlic and sauté for 1 minute. Stir in the flour, bouillon, and pepper until well-blended. Gradually stir in the milk, and cook, stirring constantly until thickened. Reduce the heat to low and stir in the cheese until melted. Pour 1 cup of cheese sauce into a 9-inch round baking dish. Place the shells in the baking dish, and cover with the remaining sauce. Bake at 350° for 20 to 25 minutes. If desired, broil for 3 to 5 minutes or until lightly browned. Serve immediately.

Veal Provençale

3 tomatoes
6 tablespoons safflower oil
3 scallions, chopped
8 veal scallopini (4 ounces each)
  Pepper to taste
6 tablespoons dry white wine
½ bunch basil

Exchange Values Per Serving:
½ Vegetable
3 Meat
1 Fat

246 Calories
(57% from Fat)
3.3gm Carbohydrates
22.8gm Protein
15.5gm Fat
116mg Cholesterol
107mg Sodium
517mg Potassium

Chop the tomatoes after removing the skin and seeds. Set aside. Heat the oil in a frypan, and sauté the scallions and veal. Add the pepper, tomatoes, wine, and basil. Cover the pan and cook over low heat until the liquid has reduced, about 5 minutes.

Vegetarian Lasagna

1 pound fresh spinach
  ■ ■ ■
10 lasagna noodles
  ■ ■ ■
2 cups fresh mushrooms, sliced
1 cup carrots, grated
½ cup onions, chopped
1 tablespoon safflower oil
1 15-ounce can whole tomatoes without skins, pureed
½ teaspoon basil
½ teaspoon rosemary
¼ teaspoon sage
¼ teaspoon oregano
  ■ ■ ■
2 cups lowfat cottage cheese
16 ounces Monterey Jack cheese, sliced
  ■ ■ ■
2 tablespoons grated Parmesan cheese

Exchange Values Per Serving:
2 Vegetable
1 Bread
2 Meat
1 Fat

284 Calories
(45% from Fat)
20.8gm Carbohydrates
19.0gm Protein
14.1gm Fat
33mg Cholesterol
463mg Sodium
481mg Potassium

*R*inse the spinach well. Cook the spinach in a covered saucepan without water except for the drops that cling to the leaves. Reduce the heat when the steam forms and cook 3 to 4 minutes more. Cook the lasagna noodles in boiling unsalted water, and drain. Cook the mushrooms, carrots, and onions in a saucepan in hot oil until tender, but not brown. Stir in the tomato and spices. Simmer for at least 20 minutes. In a sprayed baking dish layer as follows: lasagna noodles, cottage cheese, spinach, Monterey Jack cheese, and sauce mixture. Repeat the layers, reserving several cheese slices for the top. Then sprinkle the top with grated Parmesan. Bake at 375° for 30 minutes. Let the lasagna cool for 10 minutes before serving.

Spinach-Parmesan Lasagna

EIGHT SERVINGS

2 **bunches spinach**
¼ **pound mushrooms, sliced**
1 **cup lowfat cottage cheese**
¼ **teaspoon nutmeg**
⅛ **teaspoon pepper**

■ ■ ■

8 **cooked lasagna noodles**

■ ■ ■

1 **clove garlic, minced**
½ **cup sliced onion**
2 **cups pureed whole tomatoes**
½ **teaspoon basil**
½ **teaspoon oregano**

■ ■ ■

2 **tablespoons grated Parmesan cheese**

Exchange Values
Per Serving:
1 Vegetable
1 Bread
1 Meat

136 Calories
(10% from Fat)
22.3gm Carbohydrates
8.9gm Protein
1.5gm Fat
3mg Cholesterol
259mg Sodium
435mg Potassium

*S*team the spinach until limp, and then chop. Mix with the mushrooms, cottage cheese, and seasonings. Line each noodle with 2 to 3 tablespoons of this mixture, roll up, and place standing up in a shallow baking pan. Combine the remaining ingredients except the Parmesan and pour over the noodles. Sprinkle lightly with Parmesan cheese. Bake at 350° degrees for 20 minutes.

Manicotti with Eggplant-Tomato Relish

NINE SERVINGS

1 pound lean ground beef
¼ cup finely chopped onion
¼ cup finely chopped celery
½ cup tomato paste
½ cup Ricotta cheese
¼ cup fine dry seasoned bread crumbs
4 egg whites, lightly beaten
1 teaspoon minced garlic
9 manicotti shells

■ ■ ■

3 tablespoons margarine
3 tablespoons all-purpose flour
⅛ teaspoon pepper
2½ cups skim milk
¼ cup grated Parmesan cheese

■ ■ ■

1½ cups diced, peeled eggplant
2 tablespoons chopped onion
½ cup water
2 tablespoons tomato paste
2 tablespoons water
1 tablespoon liquid margarine
2 tablespoons chopped fresh parsley
2 tablespoons sliced ripe black olives
¼ teaspoon *each* oregano, thyme
¼ cup diced fresh tomato

*Exchange Values
Per Serving:*
½ Milk
1 Vegetable
2 Bread
2 Meat
1 Fat

446 Calories
(37% from Fat)
43gm Carbohydrates
26.7gm Protein
18.1gm Fat
45mg Cholesterol
297mg Sodium
600mg Potassium

*B*rown the ground beef with the onion and celery in a large skillet. Remove from the heat and stir in the tomato paste. Cool. Add the Ricotta cheese, bread crumbs, egg whites, and garlic. Meanwhile, cook the manicotti according to the package directions. Cool in a single layer on waxed paper for easier handling. Using a teaspoon, generously fill the shells with meat mixture.

Melt the margarine in a saucepan. Stir in the flour and ⅛ teaspoon of pepper. Gradually add the milk, cooking and stirring until thick and bubbly. Blend in the Parmesan cheese. Spoon 1½ cups of sauce into a greased 11x7x2-inch baking dish. Arrange the filled manicotti in the baking dish. Cover with aluminum foil and bake at 350° for 30 to 35 minutes or until hot and bubbly.

Combine the eggplant and onion in a small saucepan. Simmer in ½ cup of water for about 3 minutes or until tender. Drain. Combine the tomato paste with 2 tablespoons of water. Add to the eggplant mixture, and stir in the remaining ingredients.

To serve, spoon the manicotti onto a serving plate and serve with the remaining sauce and Eggplant-Tomato Relish.

Manicotti with Ratatouille Sauce

SIX SERVINGS

4	ounces Manicotti, uncooked
1¾	cups Ricotta cheese
1	cup shredded Mozzarella cheese
¼	cup grated Parmesan cheese
2	egg whites, lightly beaten
¼	cup chopped fresh parsley
⅛	teaspoon pepper

■ ■ ■

2	tablespoons olive oil
2	cups diced peeled eggplant
1	cup sliced onion
1	cup green pepper strips
2	cloves garlic, minced
2	cups thinly sliced zucchini
½	teaspoon *each* oregano, basil
¼	teaspoon *each* marjoram, pepper
1	15-ounce can tomato sauce
1	14½-ounce can stewed tomatoes
	Grated Parmesan cheese (optional)

Exchange Values
Per Serving:
2 Vegetable
2 Bread
2 Meat
1 Fat

392 Calories
(41% from Fat)
34.3gm Carbohydrates
25.3gm Protein
18.0gm Fat
47mg Cholesterol
890mg Sodium
877mg Potassium

Cook the manicotti according to the package directions. Drain, and cool in a single layer on wax paper for easier handling. Combine the cheeses, egg, parsley, and pepper in a mixing bowl, and spoon or pipe through a pastry tube into the manicotti. Set aside.

Sauté the eggplant, onion, green pepper, and garlic in a large saucepan for 5 minutes. Blend in the zucchini, seasonings, tomato sauce, and stewed tomatoes, and simmer uncovered for 5 minutes or until the vegetables are tender. Remove from the heat and spoon half of the mixture into a 12x7½-inch baking dish. Place the manicotti over the sauce mixture. Top with the remaining sauce mixture. Bake at 350° for 20 to 25 minutes or until hot and bubbly. Serve with Parmesan cheese, if desired (not included in analysis).

Spicy Manicotti

FOUR SERVINGS

6 manicotti shells

▪ ▪ ▪

2 cups dry curd cottage cheese
¼ cup chopped parsley
1 small onion, diced
1 egg white
¼ clove garlic, minced
¼ teaspoon Italian seasoning

▪ ▪ ▪

1 14½-ounce can whole tomatoes
1 6-ounce can tomato paste

▪ ▪ ▪

½ cup shredded lowfat cheese

*Exchange Values
Per Serving:*
2 Vegetable
1 Bread
2 Meat

245 Calories
(23% from Fat)
26.1gm Carbohydrates
22gm Protein
6.5gm Fat
21mg Cholesterol
801mg Sodium
741mg Potassium

Cook the manicotti according to the package directions, omitting salt. Drain and set aside.

Combine the cottage cheese, parsley, onion, egg white, garlic, and seasoning in a medium bowl and mix until well blended. Stuff into the shells. Puree together the whole tomatoes and tomato paste. Spoon some sauce into the bottom of the baking dish and arrange the stuffed shells over this. Cover the centers of each shell with sauce and sprinkle with shredded cheese. Cover and bake at 350° for 20 to 25 minutes.

Vegetables and Rice

Asparagus and Basil

SIX SERVINGS

2 tablespoons liquid margarine
¼ teaspoon crushed dried basil leaves
   Pepper to taste
1 teaspoon lemon juice
2 pounds cooked asparagus

*M*elt the margarine in a saucepan. Add the basil, pepper, and lemon juice. Pour over the cooked asparagus and serve hot.

Exchange Values
Per Serving:
1½ Vegetable
1 Fat

76 Calories
(45% from Fat)
7.5gm Carbohydrates
4.5gm Protein
4.4gm Fat
0mg Cholesterol
50mg Sodium
332mg Potassium

Baked Broccoli

2 **10-ounce packages frozen chopped broccoli**
1 **10¾-ounce can condensed cream of mushroom soup**
½ **cup plain lowfat yogurt**
¼ **cup egg substitute**
1 **small onion, grated**
1 **cup shredded imitation Cheddar cheese**
1 **cup cheese cracker crumbs**
¼ **cup liquid margarine**

Exchange Values Per Serving:
1 Vegetable
1 Bread
1 Meat
1 Fat

227 Calories
(47% from Fat)
18.3gm Carbohydrates
13.1gm Protein
11.8gm Fat
2mg Cholesterol
939mg Sodium
294mg Potassium

Cook the broccoli slightly. Drain, and combine with the soup, yogurt, egg substitute, onion, and cheese. Place in a 2-quart casserole. Toss the cracker crumbs with the melted margarine, and spoon over the broccoli mixture. Bake at 350° for 30 to 35 minutes.

Broccoli and Herbs

3 **pounds broccoli**
2 **cups chicken broth**
½ **cup chopped onion**
1 **teaspoon minced garlic**
1 **teaspoon marjoram**
1 **bay leaf**
½ **teaspoon Mrs. Dash mixed herbs**
2 **tablespoons liquid margarine**

Exchange Values Per Serving:
2 Vegetable
1 Fat

118 Calories
(39% from Fat)
13.7gm Carbohydrates
8.6gm Protein
5.1gm Fat
0mg Cholesterol
387mg Sodium
832mg Potassium

Wash the broccoli well and remove the leaves. Cut and prepare for cooking. Bring the chicken broth to a boil in a large skillet with a lid. Add all of the ingredients except the margarine. Cook covered for 10 to 15 minutes or until the broccoli is tender. Drain and drizzle the margarine over the spears.

Broccoli and Rice Casserole

FOUR SERVINGS

¼ cup chopped onion
1 tablespoon liquid margarine
2 10-ounce boxes chopped broccoli, cooked
1 cup rice, cooked in 2 cups water
1 10¾-ounce can cream of celery soup
½ cup skim milk
1 cup shredded imitation sharp Cheddar cheese
2 teaspoons pepper
2 tablespoons Parmesan cheese

*S*auté the onion in the margarine. Combine all of the ingredients except the Parmesan in a sprayed casserole dish. Sprinkle with Parmesan cheese. Cover and bake at 350° for 30 minutes.

Exchange Values
Per Serving:
2 Vegetable
2½ Bread
2½ Meat

422 Calories
(25% from Fat)
56.4gm Carbohydrates
24.5gm Protein
11.7gm Fat
11mg Cholesterol
1567mg Sodium
537mg Potassium

Broccoli and Rice Casserole

SIX SERVINGS

2½ cups brown rice, cooked
2 egg whites
1 small onion
1 bunch fresh broccoli
1 cup lowfat cottage cheese
½ teaspoon pepper
1 cup croutons
½ cup lowfat milk
2 tablespoons Parmesan cheese

*C*ombine the rice, egg whites, onion, broccoli, cottage cheese, pepper, croutons, and milk with a wooden spoon. Pour into a lightly sprayed casserole. Sprinkle the top with Parmesan and bake at 350° for 30 to 40 minutes until tender.

Exchange Values
Per Serving:
1 Vegetable
2 Bread
1½ Meat

258 Calories
(15% from Fat)
40.6gm Carbohydrates
17.8gm Protein
4.2gm Fat
6.3mg Cholesterol
620mg Sodium
921mg Potassium

Broccoli Casserole

2 **cups cooked rice**
2 **10-ounce packages frozen chopped broccoli**
1 **10-ounce can condensed cream of mushroom soup**
1 **cup plain lowfat yogurt**
1 **cup shredded lowfat American cheese**
1 **medium onion, chopped**
½ **cup egg substitute**

*Exchange Values
Per Serving:*
1 Vegetable
1 Bread
1 Meat

197 Calories
(27% from Fat)
22.8gm Carbohydrates
14.1gm Protein
5.9gm Fat
2mg Cholesterol
985mg Sodium
349mg Potassium

Spread the rice in the bottom of a casserole dish. Steam the broccoli in a small amount of water for 5 minutes or until crisp-tender. Spoon over the rice. Mix together the remaining ingredients and pour over the broccoli. Bake at 350° for 30 to 35 minutes. Cut into 8 equal portions.

Broccoli Turkey Casserole

2 **10-ounce packages frozen chopped broccoli**
2 **10¾-ounce cans turkey broth**
2 **cups diced, cooked turkey**
½ **teaspoon sage**
½ **cup chopped onions**
½ **cup chopped celery**
1 **egg**
2 **cups bread, cut up**
2 **tablespoons liquid margarine**

*Exchange Values
Per Serving:*
½ Vegetable
½ Bread
2 Meat
1 Fat

188 Calories
(40% from Fat)
8.6gm Carbohydrates
21.8gm Protein
7.3gm Fat
78mg Cholesterol
380mg Sodium
441mg Potassium

Toss together all of the ingredients except the melted margarine. Pour into a sprayed casserole dish and pour the margarine over the top. Cover and bake at 350° for 35 to 40 minutes. Uncover and bake an additional 15 minutes or until the vegetables are tender.

Creole Cabbage

5 cups chopped cabbage
1 large onion, chopped
1 teaspoon garlic, minced
1 green pepper, chopped
2 tablespoons margarine
1 16-ounce can tomatoes
1 teaspoon sugar
Pepper to taste
1 cup shredded imitation sharp Cheddar cheese

Exchange Values Per Serving:
2 Vegetable
1 Meat

112 Calories
(42% from Fat)
8.9gm Carbohydrates
8.5gm Protein
5.2gm Fat
0mg Cholesterol
571mg Sodium
316mg Potassium

Cook the cabbage in water for 10 minutes. Drain well and place in pan. Sauté the onions, garlic, and green pepper in the margarine. Add the tomatoes with juice, sugar, and pepper, and simmer for 5 minutes or more. Combine this mixture with the cabbage and place in a baking dish. Sprinkle with cheese and bake at 325° for about 20 minutes or until the cheese melts.

Sweet Carrots with Dill or Basil

1 pound carrots
½ cup water
1 tablespoon liquid margarine
½ cup orange juice
½ teaspoon vanilla extract
2 teaspoons dill seed or sweet basil

Exchange Values Per Serving:
2 Vegetable
¼ Fruit
½ Fat

88 Calories
(30% from Fat)
14.8gm Carbohydrates
1.4gm Protein
3.1gm Fat
0mg Cholesterol
73mg Sodium
431mg Potassium

Cut the carrots into diagonal slices. Steam or boil in ½ cup water for 10 minutes in a large saucepan. Drain and add the margarine, orange juice, vanilla, and dill or basil. Simmer 10 to 15 minutes more, until the carrots are tender.

Crumbly Cauliflower

EIGHT SERVINGS

1	head cauliflower
¼	cup liquid margarine
½	teaspoon salt substitute
½	teaspoon pepper
1	cup cheese cracker crumbs
½	cup diced green pepper
1	16-ounce can tomatoes, chopped
1	medium onion, chopped
1½	cups shredded low-calorie Cheddar cheese

*W*ash the cauliflower and remove the leaves. Break into flowerets. Cook for 5 minutes in salted water. Drain. Combine the margarine, pepper and cracker crumbs in a large mixing bowl. Stir in the green pepper, tomatoes, onion, and 1¼ cups cheese with the hot drained cauliflower. Pour into a 2-quart casserole. Sprinkle with the remaining cheese. Bake at 350° for 1 hour. Serve hot.

Exchange Values Per Serving:
2 Vegetable
½ Bread
1 Meat
1 Fat

209 Calories
(41% from Fat)
17.8gm Carbohydrates
14.1gm Protein
9.6gm Fat
1mg Cholesterol
647mg Sodium
427mg Potassium

Cheesy Scalloped Cucumbers

FOUR SERVINGS

3	slices bread
3	large cucumbers, peeled and sliced ⅓- to ½-inch thick
	Pepper to taste
	Salt substitute to taste
2	tablespoons minced onion
½	cup liquid margarine
¾	cup skim milk
1	cup grated low-calorie sharp Cheddar cheese

*C*rumble the bread into a sprayed baking dish. Arrange about half the cucumber slices over the bread crumbs and sprinkle with pepper, salt substitute, and a small amount of minced onion. Add a little margarine. Repeat the layers and pour skim milk over all. Sprinkle the top with grated Cheddar. Bake at 350° for 30 minutes or until browned.

Exchange Values Per Serving:
1 Vegetable
1 Bread
2 Meat
1 Fat

240 Calories
(33% from Fat)
22.6gm Carbohydrates
18.8gm Protein
8.7gm Fat
1mg Cholesterol
1055mg Sodium
556mg Potassium

Stuffed Eggplant

FOUR SERVINGS

1   large eggplant
½   cup water
½   teaspoon salt substitute
¼   cup chopped onion
1   tablespoon liquid margarine
1   10½-ounce can condensed cream of mushroom soup
1   teaspoon Worcestershire sauce
1   cup fine cracker crumbs
1   tablespoon chopped parsley
1½ cups water

Exchange Values
Per Serving:
2 Vegetable
2½ Bread
2 Fat

240 Calories
(37% from Fat)
33.5gm Carbohydrates
6.1gm Protein
9.8gm Fat
0mg Cholesterol
833mg Sodium
410mg Potassium

*S*lice off one side of the egg plant. Remove the pulp to within ½ inch of the skin. Dice the pulp and place in a saucepan. Add ½ cup of water and the salt substitute. Simmer until the eggplant is tender. Drain. Sauté the onion in margarine until golden brown. Stir the onion, mushroom soup, Worcestershire sauce and all of the cracker crumbs except 2 tablespoons into the eggplant pulp. Fill the eggplant shell with the mixture. Place the eggplant in a shallow baking pan. Sprinkle the top with the reserved crumbs and parsley. Pour 1½ cups of water into the baking pan. Bake at 375° for 1 hour, until piping hot.

Cajun Green Beans

SIX SERVINGS

1   pound fresh French-style green beans
    Water as needed
½   cup chopped green pepper
½   cup chopped onion
2   tablespoons margarine
1   tablespoon chopped pimiento
⅓   cup chili sauce
1   teaspoon paprika

Exchange Values
Per Serving:
1½ Vegetable
1 Fat

80 Calories
(42% from Fat)
10.5gm Carbohydrates
2gm Protein
4.1gm Fat
0mg Cholesterol
208mg Sodium
306mg Potassium

*C*ook the beans in water until tender. Drain. Sauté the green pepper, celery, and onion in margarine until tender. Add the seasonings and beans, and stir until just heated through.

French Green Beans Almondine

1 **bouillon cube**
⅓ **cup boiling water**
1 **10-ounce package French-cut green beans**
1 **tablespoon slivered almonds**
1 **tablespoon liquid margarine**

*D*issolve the bouillon cube in the boiling water. Add the green beans and boil until tender. In a separate pan sauté the almonds in margarine until brown. Drain the beans and almonds, and toss together.

Exchange Values Per Serving:
1 Vegetable
1 Fat

70 Calories
(65% from Fat)
4.9gm Carbohydrates
1.6gm Protein
5.4gm Fat
0mg Cholesterol
257mg Sodium
100mg Potassium

French Green Bean and Rice Casserole

1 **large onion, chopped**
4 **teaspoons liquid margarine**
½ **cup uncooked rice**
1 **16-ounce can French-style green beans**
⅛ **teaspoon pepper**
1 **16-ounce can tomatoes**
⅓ **cup water**
1 **teaspoon Mrs. Dash seasonings**

*S*auté the onions in margarine until brown. Add the rice, tomatoes, green beans, and other ingredients. Cook, covered, for 30 minutes.

Exchange Values Per Serving:
2 Vegetable
1½ Bread
1 Fat

183 Calories
(22% from Fat)
32.9gm Carbohydrates
4.3gm Protein
4.4gm Fat
0mg Cholesterol
536mg Sodium
440mg Potassium

Apples and Onions Side Dish

FOUR SERVINGS

4 teaspoons liquid margarine
2 onions, peeled and sliced
4 medium-size firm apples, cored and sliced
   Pepper to taste
   Salt substitute to taste
½ teaspoon freshly squeezed lemon juice

*H*eat the margarine in a large skillet. Add the onions and apples, and cook, turning occasionally with a spatula, until the apples and onions are tender. Season to taste. Stir in the lemon juice. Serve hot as a side dish.

Exchange Values Per Serving:
1 Vegetable
1 Fruit
1 Fat

131 Calories
(30% from Fat)
24.2gm Carbohydrates
1gm Protein
4.4gm Fat
0mg Cholesterol
39mg Sodium
564mg Potassium

Baked Italian Onions

SIX SERVINGS

6 onions
6 tablespoons low-calorie Italian salad dressing (not creamy)
¾ cup Parmesan cheese

*P*eel and wash the onions. Slice the ends evenly so they sit straight. Score each onion in a cross like fashion leaving the outer ring intact. Place in an aluminum foil square that has been coated with coating spray. Pull the foil up around the onion leaving the top exposed, not sealed (tulip-fashioned). Spoon one tablespoon of salad dressing over the onion and sprinkle the top with 2 tablespoons of Parmesan cheese. Bake at 350° for 1 hour.

Exchange Values Per Serving:
1 Vegetable
1 Meat

101 Calories
(30% from Fat)
12.5gm Carbohydrates
5.8gm Protein
3.4gm Fat
8mg Cholesterol
350mg Sodium
234mg Potassium

Black-Eyed Peas and Wild Rice

FOUR SERVINGS

1 cup uncooked wild rice
2 cups water
1 tablespoon soy sauce
1 bunch green onions, chopped
1 cube vegetable bouillon
1 10-ounce box frozen black-eyed peas
2 tablespoons liquid margarine

*B*ring the first 5 ingredients to a boil, reduce the heat and cook for 20 minutes. Add the peas and margarine to the rice mixture and bring back to a boil, reduce the heat and cook for an additional 15 to 20 minutes.

Exchange Values Per Serving:
½ Vegetable
1½ Bread
½ Fat

152 Calories
(20% from Fat)
24.8gm Carbohydrates
6.6gm Protein
3.4gm Fat
0mg Cholesterol
224mg Sodium
242mg Potassium

Stuffed Peppers

EIGHT SERVINGS

4 large bell peppers
1½ pounds 85% or leaner ground beef
1 cup chopped onions
1 tablespoon minced parsley
½ teaspoon oregano
1 6-ounce can tomato paste
½ cup water
¾ cup shredded lowfat cheese

*C*ut the tops off the bell peppers and remove the seeds. Hollow out and wash well. Place in a baking pan. Brown the ground beef with the onion, parsley, and oregano. Add the tomato paste and water, and stir well. Spoon into the bell peppers and sprinkle with shredded cheese. Bake at 350° for 15 to 20 minutes. Remove and serve surrounded with white rice (not included in analysis).

Exchange Values Per Serving:
½ Vegetable
3 Meat
1 Fat

299 Calories
(59% from Fat)
8.8gm Carbohydrates
21.7gm Protein
19.5gm Fat
64mg Cholesterol
406mg Sodium
557mg Potassium

Baked Fluffy Potatoes

EIGHT SERVINGS

4 large Idaho baking potatoes
1 cup plain lowfat yogurt
1 tablespoon liquid margarine
½ teaspoon diced thyme
½ teaspoon diced oregano
1 cup Parmesan cheese

*B*ake the potatoes at 400° for 30 minutes or until tender. Remove from the oven and slice each in half. Hollow the potato out and retain the skins. Whip together the potato, yogurt, margarine, thyme, and oregano. Spoon back into the potato skins. Place on a cooking sheet and sprinkle each with Parmesan cheese. Place back in the oven and bake until golden brown.

Exchange Values Per Serving:
  2 Bread
  1 Meat

210 Calories
(21% from Fat)
32.8gm Carbohydrates
9.1gm Protein
5.0gm Fat
10mg Cholesterol
230mg Sodium
997mg Potassium

Cheesy Whipped Potatoes

EIGHT SERVINGS

3 pounds cooked, peeled and whipped potatoes
3 tablespoons liquid margarine
6 ounces lowfat cottage cheese
1 green pepper, chopped
½ cup grated imitation Cheddar cheese
¼ cup grated Parmesan cheese

*W*hip the cooked potatoes with the margarine, cottage cheese, pepper, and imitation Cheddar cheese. Place in a baking dish and top with Parmesan cheese. Bake at 350° for 30 minutes, until golden brown.

Exchange Values Per Serving:
  2 Bread
  1 Meat
  1 Fat

230 Calories
(26% from Fat)
32.3gm Carbohydrates
11.1gm Protein
6.7gm Fat
4mg Cholesterol
406mg Sodium
974mg Potassium

Stuffed Baked Potatoes

TWELVE SERVINGS

6 **Idaho baking potatoes**
¼ **cup liquid margarine**
1 **tablespoon minced onion**
1 **cup plain lowfat yogurt**
   Paprika
   Pepper
2 **tablespoons cheese cracker crumbs**

*Exchange Values
Per Serving:*
1 Bread
1 Fat

120 Calories
(32% from Fat)
17.8gm Carbohydrates
3.3gm Protein
4.3gm Fat
1.2mg Cholesterol
64mg Sodium
533mg Potassium

*B*ake the potatoes until tender. When they are done, split them lengthwise and scoop the potatoes out of the shells. While still hot, whip the potatoes with the margarine, yogurt, and seasonings to taste. Spoon the mixture back into the shells. Sprinkle the tops with the cracker crumbs. Return to the oven and bake at 350° for an additional 10 minutes.

Fruity Sweet Potatoes

SIX SERVINGS

4 **medium sweet potatoes, unpeeled**
¼ **cup pineapple juice**
2 **tablespoons oil**
1 **tablespoon chopped pineapple**
   Pinch cinnamon, nutmeg, and allspice

*Exchange Values
Per Serving:*
2 Bread
1 Fat

166 Calories
(27% from Fat)
29.2gm Carbohydrates
1.9gm Protein
4.9gm Fat
0mg Cholesterol
15mg Sodium
247mg Potassium

*B*oil the potatoes until tender, about 30 minutes, and remove the skins. Mash the pulp. Add the fruit juice and oil, and whip until fluffy. Add the chopped pineapple and spices, and transfer to an oiled 1-quart baking dish. Bake at 375° for 30 minutes or until lightly browned.

Cheesy Scalloped Potatoes

EIGHT SERVINGS

2½ cups skim milk
6 medium potatoes
¼ cup diced onions
¼ cup diced celery
  Paprika
3 tablespoons all-purpose flour
3 tablespoons plain lowfat yogurt
⅛ teaspoon pepper
2 tablespoons Parmesan cheese
2 tablespoons liquid margarine

Exchange Values Per Serving:
½ Milk
1 Bread
½ Fat

144 Calories
(23% from Fat)
21.9gm Carbohydrates
5.6gm Protein
3.6gm Fat
3mg Cholesterol
103mg Sodium
625mg Potassium

Scald the skim milk, set aside and allow to cool to lukewarm. Place a layer of cut-up potatoes in the bottom of a baking pan. Sprinkle with half the onion, celery and paprika.

To the milk add the flour, yogurt, and pepper. Pour half on the first layer of potatoes and sprinkle with Parmesan cheese. Repeat the layers of potatoes, celery, and onion. Sprinkle with paprika, and cover with the remaining yogurt sauce. Sprinkle with Parmesan. Dot the top of the potatoes with margarine. Cover and bake at 350° for 30 minutes. Uncover and bake further for 50 minutes or until the potatoes are tender.

Summer Squash Casserole

FOUR SERVINGS

3 to 4 medium yellow squash, sliced about ¼-inch thick
3 medium tomatoes, sliced about ¼-inch thick
½ cup thinly sliced onions
½ cup plain lowfat yogurt
½ cup shredded imitation sharp Cheddar cheese
2 teaspoons Mrs. Dash mixed herbs

Exchange Values Per Serving:
2 Vegetable
1 Meat

120 Calories
(22% from Fat)
14.6gm Carbohydrates
10.9gm Protein
2.9gm Fat
2mg Cholesterol
457mg Sodium
542mg Potassium

Layer half the vegetables in a sprayed 2-quart casserole. Spread the yogurt over the vegetables. Combine the cheese and seasonings. Sprinkle half the cheese mixture over the yogurt. Top with the remaining vegetables and then the cheese mixture. Bake at 350° for 30 minutes.

Squash and Apple Dish

FOUR SERVINGS

2 butternut, buttercup, or acorn squash
2 large tart apples, cored and sliced
½ onion, chopped
   Cinnamon
   Pepper to taste
2 teaspoons liquid margarine

Exchange Values Per Serving:
  1 Fruit
  1 Bread
  ½ Fat

121 Calories
(18% from Fat)
26.9gm Carbohydrates
1.3gm Protein
2.4gm Fat
0mg Cholesterol
22mg Sodium
506mg Potassium

*S*plit the squash in half. Scoop out the seeds and place cut side down in a greased shallow baking dish. Pour in hot water to a depth of ½-inch. Bake at 350° until partly tender, about 20 minutes for butternut or buttercup squash, 30 to 45 minutes for acorn squash.

Turn the squash cut sides up. Arrange a quarter of the apple slices and some of the onion in the cup of each squash half. Sprinkle lightly with cinnamon, and pepper to taste. Sprinkle ¼ teaspoon of the sugar over each half and dot with ½ teaspoon margarine. Add hot water to the dish, if necessary, to bring the depth to ½-inch again. Return to the 350° oven and bake for 20 to 30 minutes longer, until both the squash and the apple are tender.

Spaghetti Squash and Vegetables

EIGHT SERVINGS

1 medium spaghetti squash
6 large tomatoes, cut up
1 large onion, coarsely chopped
1 tablespoon Italian seasoning
2 cups mixed fresh vegetables such as broccoli, cauliflower, and
   carrots

Exchange Values Per Serving:
  2 Vegetable

57 Calories
(9% from Fat)
12.7gm Carbohydrates
2.8gm Protein
0.6gm Fat
0mg Cholesterol
26mg Sodium
536mg Potassium

*S*plit the spaghetti squash in half. Scoop out the seeds and place cut side down on a greased baking sheet. Bake at 350° for 35 to 45 minutes. Scoop out with a fork, it will come out in strands like spaghetti. Drain if needed. Set aside.

Bring the tomatoes, onion, and seasoning to a boil, then reduce the heat to a simmer. Cook for approximately 25 minutes. Before serving, add the cooked vegetables to the sauce. Serve over the spaghetti squash.

Broiled Tomatoes

SIX SERVINGS

6 small fresh tomatoes, not too ripe
½ cup cracker crumbs
½ cup grated Parmesan cheese
⅛ cup minced parsley
¼ cup liquid margarine

Slice the tomatoes ½-inch thick, discarding the ends. Place on broiler pan. Mix the remaining ingredients and place an equal portion of the mixture on the top of each tomato. Broil for 5 minut until hot, and serve immediately.

Exchange Values Per Serving:
1 Vegetable
½ Bread
2 Fat

156 Calories
(59% from Fat)
11.6gm Carbohydrates
5.2gm Protein
10.2gm Fat
6mg Cholesterol
273mg Sodium
245mg Potassium

Mexican Cherry Tomatoes

FOUR SERVINGS

20 cherry tomatoes
2 medium avocados
2 teaspoons Worcestershire sauce
1 tablespoon lemon juice
1 tablespoon minced onion
6 to 10 drops Tabasco sauce
2 tablespoons plain lowfat yogurt
¼ teaspoon salt substitute

Slice the tops off the cherry tomatoes. Hollow out the inside of the small tomatoes and reserve the pulp. Turn the tomatoes over and drain for 20 minutes. Peel the avocados, then mash in a food processor. Mix the remaining ingredients including the pulp from the tomatoes until light and smooth. Fill the tomatoes with the mixture.

Exchange Values Per Serving:
1 Vegetable
3 Fat

183 Calories
(77% from Fat)
11.9gm Carbohydrates
3.1gm Protein
15.6gm Fat
0.4mg Cholesterol
47mg Sodium
790mg Potassium

Steamed Vegetables

SIX SERVINGS

5   large carrots, peeled
4   medium new potatoes, quartered
12 Brussels sprouts, halved
1   tablespoon margarine, melted
1   tablespoon fresh lemon juice
⅛   teaspoon pepper

*P*lace the carrots and potatoes in a steamer over 1 to 2 inches of boiling water. Cover and cook for 6 minutes. Add the Brussels sprouts, cover, and continue cooking for 5 to 7 minutes or until the vegetables are tender. Combine the margarine, lemon juice, and pepper. Toss with the steamed vegetables. Serve with Poached Beef Tenderloin (see page 159).

Exchange Values Per Serving:
1½ Vegetable
1 Bread
½ Fat

132 Calories
(15% from Fat)
25.9gm Carbohydrates
4.0gm Protein
2.2gm Fat
0mg Cholesterol
55mg Sodium
841mg Potassium

Baked Zucchini and Cheese

FOUR SERVINGS

2   medium zucchini, sliced very thin
1   egg
1   teaspoon seasoned mustard
⅛   teaspoon ground white pepper
⅛   teaspoon ground nutmeg
1   small Vidalia onion, sliced very thin
1   tomato, sliced thin
⅓   cup Parmesan cheese

*D*rain and dry the zucchini. Combine the egg, mustard, pepper, nutmeg, and onion. Add the zucchini and stir gently. Pour into a lightly oiled casserole dish. Place the tomato slices on top and sprinkle with Parmesan. Cover and bake at 350° for 30 to 40 minutes or until a fork inserts easily.

Exchange Values Per Serving:
1 Vegetable
1 Meat

71 Calories
(43% from Fat)
5.3gm Carbohydrates
5.3gm Protein
3.4gm Fat
64mg Cholesterol
144mg Sodium
271mg Potassium

Zucchini Bake

EIGHT SERVINGS

4 large zucchini, sliced ½-inch thick
1 cup shredded lowfat Cheddar cheese
⅓ cup skim milk
½ cup plain lowfat yogurt
¼ cup flavored dry bread crumbs

*L*ayer the zucchini in a baking casserole dish. Mix ½ cup of the cheddar cheese, the skim milk, and yogurt together and pour over the zucchini. Sprinkle the top with Cheddar cheese and bread crumbs. Bake at 350° for 40 to 45 minutes, or until the zucchini is easily pierced with a fork and the top of the casserole is lightly browned.

Exchange Values Per Serving:
1 Meat
1 Vegetable

86 Calories
(26% from Fat)
7.2gm Carbohydrates
9.4gm Protein
2.5gm Fat
1mg Cholesterol
482mg Sodium
278mg Potassium

Zucchini Casserole

FOUR SERVINGS

6 zucchini squash
3 ounces plain lowfat yogurt
⅛ teaspoon garlic powder
⅛ cup minced onion
½ cup bread crumbs
⅛ teaspoon paprika
2 tablespoons Parmesan cheese

*S*lice the squash into 2-inch pieces. Cook in a small amount of boiling water for 8 to 10 minutes. Drain the zucchini well, and mix in the yogurt, garlic, and onion. Place in a sprayed casserole and top with bread crumbs and Parmesan cheese. Sprinkle with paprika. Bake at 350° for 30 minutes.

Exchange Values Per Serving:
1 Vegetable
½ Bread
½ Fat

92 Calories
(14% from Fat)
16.4gm Carbohydrates
4.3gm Protein
1.5gm Fat
4mg Cholesterol
139mg Sodium
502mg Potassium

Zucchini-Ricotta Casserole

FOUR SERVINGS

1 small onion, diced
½ pound zucchini, chopped
1 tablespoon liquid margarine
3 tablespoons all-purpose flour
Dash salt and pepper
Dash paprika
¾ cup egg substitute
1 pound part skim Ricotta cheese
½ cup grated lowfat cheese
Dash nutmeg

Exchange Values
Per Serving:
3 Meat
1 Fat
1 Vegetable

220 Calories
(49% from Fat)
9.6gm Carbohydrates
18.0gm Protein
12.0gm Fat
35.7mg Cholesterol
283mg Sodium
339mg Potassium

*S*auté the onion and zucchini in margarine. Stir in flour. Add the salt, pepper, and paprika. Remove from the heat, add the remaining ingredients, and mix well. Bake in a 1½-quart casserole dish at 350° for 35 to 40 minutes.

Oriental Oat Pilaf

SIX SERVINGS

1 tablespoon liquid margarine
1 cup sliced mushrooms
½ cup chopped red pepper
½ cup sliced green onions
½ cup chopped celery
1¾ cups quick cooking or old-fashioned oats, dry
2 egg whites
2 tablespoons soy sauce
1 cup chicken broth
1 6-ounce package frozen pea pods, thawed

Exchange Values
Per Serving:
1 Vegetable
1 Bread
½ Fat

143 Calories
(24% from Fat)
20.2gm Carbohydrates
7.4gm Protein
3.8gm Fat
0.3mg Cholesterol
452mg Sodium
317mg Potassium

*M*elt the margarine in a skillet over medium heat. Add the mushrooms, pepper, onions, and celery, and sauté for 2 to 3 minutes. Mix the oats, egg whites, and soy sauce. Coat the oats well, then add to the vegetable mixture. Cook for an additional 5 minutes or until lightly browned. Add the chicken broth and pea pods, and cook until the liquid is absorbed and the vegetables are tender.

Golden Mediterranean Pilaf

SIX SERVINGS

3   cups chicken broth
1½   cups uncooked long grain white rice
4   tablespoons safflower oil
½   cup seedless golden raisins
½   teaspoon turmeric
½   teaspoon curry powder
1   tablespoon soy sauce

*Exchange Values
Per Serving:*
1 Fruit
2 Bread
2 Fat

316 Calories
(29% from Fat)
49.7gm Carbohydrates
6.2gm Protein
10.1gm Fat
0mg Cholesterol
530mg Sodium
252mg Potassium

*B*ring the chicken broth to a boil in a 1 quart saucepan. In another medium saucepan, combine the rice, safflower oil, raisins, turmeric, curry, and soy sauce. Pour the chicken broth over the rice mix. Cover and cook over low heat for 20 minutes or until all of the liquid is absorbed and the rice is tender.

Old-Fashioned Macaroni and Cheese

SIX SERVINGS

1½   cups skim milk
1½   tablespoons all-purpose flour
1½   tablespoons liquid margarine
¾   cup grated lowfat American cheese
2   cups macaroni, cooked and drained
¼   cup cheese cracker crumbs
      Pepper
      Paprika

*Exchange Values
Per Serving:*
1 Bread
1 Meat
1 Fat

184 Calories
(26% from Fat)
21.5gm Carbohydrates
12.0gm Protein
5.4gm Fat
1mg Cholesterol
532mg Sodium
163mg Potassium

*C*ombine the milk, flour, and margarine to make a white sauce. Return the sauce to low heat. Add the grated cheese, stirring constantly. Cook until the cheese has melted and the sauce boils. Remove from the heat. Alternate layers of macaroni and cheese sauce in a nonstick baking dish. Cover the top with cheese cracker crumbs.

Sprinkle with pepper and paprika for taste. Bake at 375° until the mixture bubbles and the crumbs turn brown.

Orange Curried Rice and Mushrooms

SIX SERVINGS

½ cup chopped onion
½ cup sliced mushrooms
¼ cup liquid margarine
2 teaspoons curry powder
1 cup uncooked rice
1 cup orange jucie
1 cup chicken broth

*S*auté the onions and mushrooms in margarine until soft. Stir in the curry powder and rice. Cook and stir for 2 minutes. Add the remaining ingredients and stir with a fork. Bring to a boil. Lower the heat, cover, and simmer for 20 minutes.

*Exchange Values
Per Serving:*
2 Bread
1½ Fat

*219 Calories
(57% from Fat)*
32.1gm Carbohydrates
3.7gm Protein
8.2gm Fat
0mg Cholesterol
219mg Sodium
201mg Potassium

Applesauce Cake

TWELVE SERVINGS

¼ cup liquid margarine
¼ cup oil
4 tablespoons sugar
1 teaspoon baking powder
¼ teaspoon baking soda
1 cup unsweetened applesauce
2 cups all-purpose flour
¼ cup egg substitute
1 teaspoon cinnamon
¼ teaspoon nutmeg
⅛ teaspoon cloves
¾ cup raisins
¾ cup chopped nuts
1 teaspoon vanilla extract

*Exchange Values
Per Serving:*
2 Bread
2 Fat

251 Calories
(48% from Fat)
30.0gm Carbohydrates
4.1gm Protein
13.4gm Fat
0mg Cholesterol
91mg Sodium
163mg Potassium

Combine all of the ingredients and mix well. Pour into a prepared bundt pan. Bake at 350° for 1 to 1½ hours or until done.

Bread Pudding with Raisins

TWO SERVINGS

2 slices day old bread, cubed
½ cup raisins
2 cups skim milk
½ cup egg substitute
2 tablespoons sugar
1 teaspoon cinnamon
1 teaspoon vanilla extract
¼ teaspoon nutmeg

Exchange Values
Per Serving:
1 Milk
2 Fruit
1 Bread
1 Meat

375 Calories
(9% from Fat)
67.8gm Carbohydrates
19.2gm Protein
3.5gm Fat
6mg Cholesterol
370mg Sodium
914mg Potassium

Combine the bread cubes and raisins in a 1½-quart baking dish. Combine the remaining ingredients and pour over the bread and raisins. Stir to combine.

Set the dish in a shallow pan. Pour hot water in the pan to a depth of 1 inch. Bake at 350° for 45 to 55 minutes or until a knife inserted in the pudding comes out clean.

Classic Sugar-Free Fruitcake

SIXTEEN SERVINGS

½ cup rum
1 6-ounce can orange juice concentrate, thawed
1 cup cranberries, chopped

■ ■ ■

1 8-ounce package pitted dates, chopped
1 cup chopped pecans
1 tablespoon grated orange rind
1 tablespoon vanilla extract
2 eggs, lightly beaten (egg substitute can also be used)
1 8-ounce can unsweetened pineapple tidbits, drained

■ ■ ■

2 cups all-purpose flour
1¼ teaspoons baking soda
½ teaspoon cinnamon

Exchange Values
Per Serving:
1 Fruit
1 Bread
1½ Fat

233 Calories
(30% from Fat)
30.5gm Carbohydrates
3.6gm Protein
7.7gm Fat
29mg Cholesterol
74mg Sodium
251mg Potassium

½ teaspoon ground nutmeg
¼ teaspoon allspice
■ ■ ■
   Vegetable cooking spray
■ ■ ■
½ cup rum
½ cup orange juice

Combine ½ cup of rum, the orange juice concentrate, and chopped cranberries and allow to stand for 1 hour. Combine the dates, pecans, orange rinds, vanilla, eggs, and pineapple. Add to the cranberry mix and stir. Combine the flour, soda, and spices. Add to the fruit mixture and stir well. Spoon the batter into a prepared, sprayed bundt pan. Bake at 325° for 45 minutes or until the cake tests done. Remove from the pan when it has cooled for 20 minutes.

Place several layers of cheesecloth over the top of the cake. Combine ½ cup of rum and ½ cup of orange juice and pour over the cloth. Allow to sit. Wrap in wax or plastic wrap and then in foil and store in a cool dry place for 1 week.

Light and Easy Poundcake

TEN SERVINGS

1   10¾-ounce frozen Sara Lee Original Pound Cake
2½ cups strawberry sherbet
5   fresh strawberries
2   kiwi fruit, sliced

Slice the frozen pound cake vertically into 5 slices, 1½-inches thick. Cut each slice in half diagonally. Top each slice with a ¼ cup scoop of sherbet, half of a strawberry, and 1 slice of kiwi fruit. Serve immediately.

Exchange Values
Per Serving:
1 Fruit
1 Bread
1½ Fat

209 Calories
(39% from Fat)
30.9gm Carbohydrates
2.3gm Protein
9.4gm Fat
62.8mg Cholesterol
128mg Sodium
128mg Potassium

Apple-Apricot Pie

4 tablespoons sugar
2 tablespoons cornstarch
2 tablespoons all-purpose flour
2 teaspoons grated lemon rind
3 tablespoons orange juice
1 teaspoon cinnamon
½ teaspoon nutmeg

■ ■ ■

1 cup chopped apricots
8 large apples, peeled, cored, and sliced

■ ■ ■

1 9-inch unbaked pie crust
   Streusel topping (see recipe on p. 196)

Exchange Values
Per Serving:
2 Fruit
1½ Bread
1½ Fat

287 Calories
(25% from Fat)
54.2gm Carbohydrates
2.7gm Protein
8.0gm Fat
0mg Cholesterol
125mg Sodium
351mg Potassium

*C*ombine the dry ingredients and mix thoroughly. Add the fruit and toss until well coated. Pour into the pie crust. Sprinkle the Streusel topping over the pie. Bake at 425° for 15 minutes, and reduce the temperature to 350° for an additional 45 minutes. Streusel topping not included in this analysis.

Apple-Cranberry Cobbler

3 cups peeled, chopped cooking apples
2 cups cranberries
¼ cup sugar
¼ cup apple juice
¼ cup all-purpose flour
1 tablespoon lemon juice
1 teaspoon cinnamon
½ teaspoon nutmeg

■ ■ ■

½ cup liquid margarine
1½ cups uncooked oatmeal

Exchange Values
Per Serving:
1 Fruit
1½ Bread
4 Fat

323 Calories
(55% from Fat)
35.1gm Carbohydrates
4.5gm Protein
19.6gm Fat

⅓ **cup all-purpose flour**
½ **cup chopped pecans**

0mg Cholesterol
113mg Sodium
191mg Potassium

Combine the apples, cranberries, sugar, apple juice, ¼ cup of flour, the lemon juice, and spices. Set aside. Combine the margarine, oatmeal, ⅓ cup of flour, and the pecans in a large bowl. Reserve ¼ cup of the mixture, and press the rest into the bottom and sides of a 9-inch pie plate. Add the apple and cranberry mixture. Sprinkle the top with the reserved oatmeal mix. Bake at 350° for 45 minutes. The cobbler should be bubbly when done.

Dutch Apple Pie

EIGHT SERVINGS

1¾ **pounds medium cooking apples**
3 **tablespoons orange juice**
1 **tablespoon cornstarch**
½ **teaspoon cinnamon**
¼ **teaspoon nutmeg**
2 **tablespoons fructose**

　　■ ■ ■

1 **9-inch pie crust**

　　■ ■ ■

½ **cup all-purpose flour**
3 **tablespoons liquid margarine**
¼ **teaspoon cinnamon**

Exchange Values
Per Serving:
1 Fruit
1 Bread
2 Fat

244 Calories
(39% from Fat)
35.9gm Carbohydrates
2.4gm Protein
10.8gm Fat
0mg Cholesterol
167mg Sodium
166mg Potassium

Combine the apples, orange juice, cornstarch, ½ teaspoon of cinnamon, nutmeg, and fructose. Blend together well, and pour into an uncooked 9-inch pie crust. Combine the flour, margarine, and ¼ teaspoon cinnamon to make a crumbly topping, and sprinkle over the pie. Bake at 350° for 1 hour.

Dutch Peach Pie

TEN SERVINGS

⅛ teaspoon allspice
⅛ teaspoon cinnamon
2 tablespoons all-purpose flour
1 tablespoon cornstarch

■ ■ ■

1 6-ounce can frozen orange juice concentrate
¾ cup water

■ ■ ■

12 peaches, peeled and sliced

■ ■ ■

1 9-inch unbaked pie crust
Streusel topping (see recipe on p. 196)

Exchange Values
Per Serving:
1 Fruit
1 Bread
1 Fat

197 Calories
(27% from Fat)
34.7gm Carbohydrates
3.1gm Protein
6.0gm Fat
0mg Cholesterol
100mg Sodium
436mg Potassium

Combine the dry ingredients in a bowl and stir in the orange juice and water. Add the peaches and mix thoroughly until well coated. Pour into the pie crust. Sprinkle the Streusel topping over the pie. Bake at 425° for 15 minutes, and reduce the temperature to 350° for an additional 45 minutes. Streusel topping not included in this analysis.

Cherry Supreme Cheesecake

EIGHT SERVINGS

1 8-ounce package reduced-calorie cream cheese
8 packets artificial sweetener
1 teaspoon vanilla extract
1 tablespoon skim milk

■ ■ ■

1 9-inch graham cracker pie shell

■ ■ ■

2 16-ounce cans tart cherries packed in water
3 tablespoons cornstarch
8 packets artificial sweetener

Exchange Values
Per Serving:
1 Fruit
1 Bread
2 Fat

224 Calories
(39% from Fat)
32.3gm Carbohydrates
3.4gm Protein

¼ **teaspoon almond extract**
2 **drops red food coloring**

9.6gm Fat
22.3mg Cholesterol
197mg Sodium
241mg Potassium

*C*ombine the cream cheese, artificial sweetener, vanilla, and milk in a food processor. Process until light and creamy. Pour into the pie shell and chill until firm. Combine the cherries, cornstarch, and remaining sweetener in the top of a double boiler, and gently heat over the water until the mixture thickens. Remove from the heat and add the almond exract and red food coloring. Cool, and spread over the cheese layer.

Baked Pumpkin Pie

EIGHT SERVINGS

2 **packets artificial sweetener**
½ **teaspoon cinnamon**
½ **teaspoon ginger**
½ **teaspoon nutmeg**
 Pinch ground cloves
1½ **cups canned pumpkin**
1 **teaspoon vanilla extract**
1½ **cups evaporated skim milk**
½ **teaspoon orange rind**
3 **egg whites, slightly beaten**
¼ **cup brandy (optional, not in analysis)**
1 **9-inch unbaked pie crust**

*Exchange Values
Per Serving:*
½ Milk
1 Bread
1½ Fat

184 Calories
(37% from Fat)
21.9gm Carbohydrates
7.2gm Protein
7.5gm Fat
2mg Cholesterol
201mg Sodium
305mg Potassium

*C*ombine the sweetener, cinnamon, ginger, nutmeg, and cloves. Stir in the pumpkin. Add the vanilla, evaporated milk, orange rind, and egg whites. Beat with an electric mixer until smooth. Fold in the brandy, if used. Pour into the pie crust and bake at 450° for 10 minutes. Reduce the oven to 325° and bake until a knife inserted in the center comes out clean, about 45 minutes.

Pumpkin Pie in a Graham Cracker Crust

EIGHT SERVINGS

1 ¼-ounce package unflavored gelatin
1 teaspoon ground ginger
½ teaspoon nutmeg
   Pinch cloves
½ cup egg substitute
1 13-ounce can evaporated skim milk
1 1-pound can pumpkin
8 packets sugar substitute
1 9-inch graham cracker crust

Exchange Values Per Serving:
½ Milk
1½ Bread
1 Fat

184 Calories
(29% from Fat)
25.9gm Carbohydrates
7.7gm Protein
6.0gm Fat
10mg Cholesterol
222mg Sodium
380mg Potassium

Mix the gelatin and spices in a medium saucepan. Beat the egg substitute and milk together and pour into the dry ingredients. Let stand for 1 minute. Stir over low heat until the gelatin is dissolved, about 10 minutes. Blend in the pumpkin and sugar substitute. Pour the mixture into a graham cracker crust and chill until firm.

Streusel Topping

EIGHT SERVINGS

1 cup all-purpose flour
1 teaspoon cinnamon
½ cup liquid margarine
1 tablespoon sugar

Exchange Values Per Serving:
1 Bread
2 Fat

163 Calories
(63% from Fat)
13.5gm Carbohydrates
1.8gm Protein
11.4gm Fat
0mg Cholesterol
132mg Sodium
21mg Potassium

Combine all of the ingredients until the mixture resembles coarse crumbs. Sprinkle over any fruit pie before baking.

Bavarian Whipped Strawberry Pie

EIGHT SERVINGS

1   3-ounce package sugar-free strawberry gelatin
1   cup boiling water
½   cup cold water
1   tablespoon lemon juice
1   6-ounce container nondairy whipping topping, unthawed
1   pint fresh strawberries, chopped to make 1 cup (keep some for garnish)
1   baked 9-inch pie crust

Dissolve the gelatin in boiling water. Add the cold water and lemon juice. Chill until slightly thickened. Fold together the gelatin mix and the nondairy topping, and blend well. Fold in the strawberries. Pour the mixture into the pie shell and chill until firm, about 3 hours. Garnish with the reserved strawberries.

Exchange Values Per Serving:
1 Bread
2½ Fat

198 Calories
(58% from Fat)
18.4gm Carbohydrates
2.9gm Protein
12.7gm Fat
0mg Cholesterol
135mg Sodium
80mg Potassium

Graham Cracker Crust

EIGHT SERVINGS

4   tablespoons liquid margarine
1¼   cups finely crumbled graham crackers
¼   teaspoon cinnamon

Melt the margarine and mix with the graham cracker crumbs and cinnamon. Press firmly into a 9-inch pie pan on the sides and the bottom. Bake at 350 for 5 minutes.

Exchange Values Per Serving:
1 Bread
1 Fat

115 Calories
(54% from Fat)
11.8gm Carbohydrates
1.2gm Protein
6.8gm Fat
0mg Cholesterol
144mg Sodium
68mg Potassium

Oat Bran Pie Crust

EIGHT SERVINGS

1 cup whole wheat flour
½ cup oat bran cereal
¼ cup safflower oil
3 tablespoons sugar-free lemon lime soda

Combine the flour and bran. Stir in the oil and crumble by hand while adding the soda. Form into a ball and roll out between two sheets of wax paper. Place in a lightly oiled pie pan and prick with a fork.

Exchange Values
Per Serving:
1 Bread
1½ Fat

138 Calories
(47% from Fat)
16gm Carbohydrates
3.9gm Protein
7.6gm Fat
0mg Cholesterol
2mg Sodium
106mg Potassium

Apricot Cookies

SIXTEEN COOKIES

½ cup liquid margarine
¼ cup sugar
¼ cup sugar-free apricot preserves
¼ cup orange juice (100%)
¼ cup water
1 teaspoon vanilla extract
¼ cup egg substitute
2 cups all-purpose flour
2 teaspoons baking powder

Combine all of the ingredients in a large bowl. Chill for 2 hours. Roll into balls and place on a cookie sheet, press down and flatten slightly. Bake at 350° for 10-12 minutes.

Exchange Values
Per Cookie:
1 Bread
1 Fat

124 Calories
(44% from Fat)
15.1gm Carbohydrates
2.2gm Protein
6.0gm Fat
0mg Cholesterol
101mg Sodium
52mg Potassium

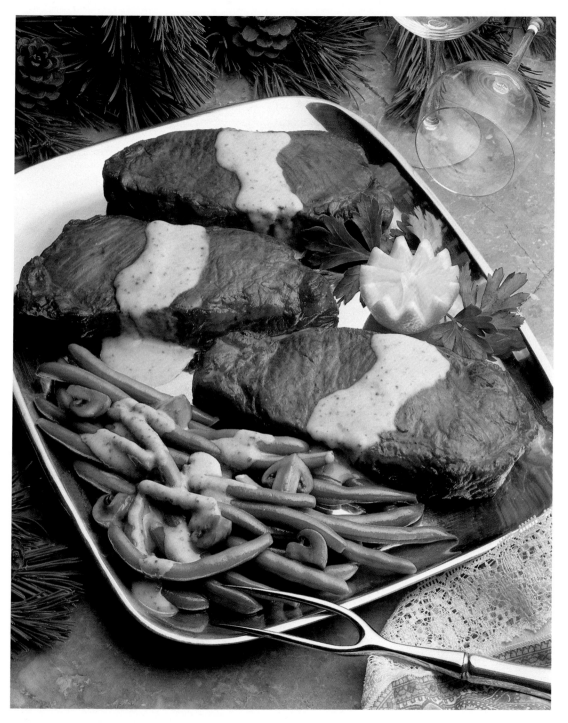

Holiday Beef Steaks with Vegetable Sauté and Hot Mustard Sauce

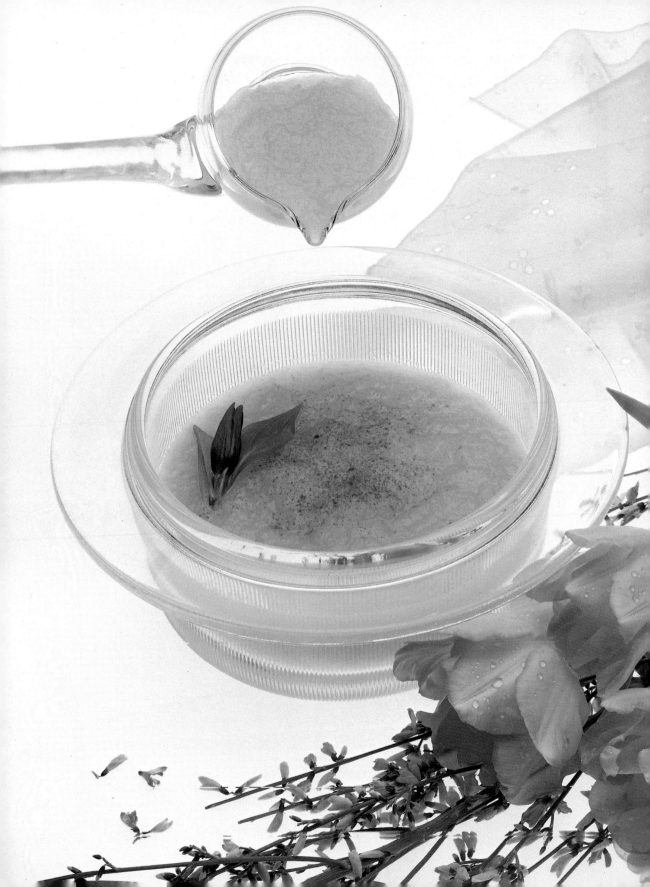

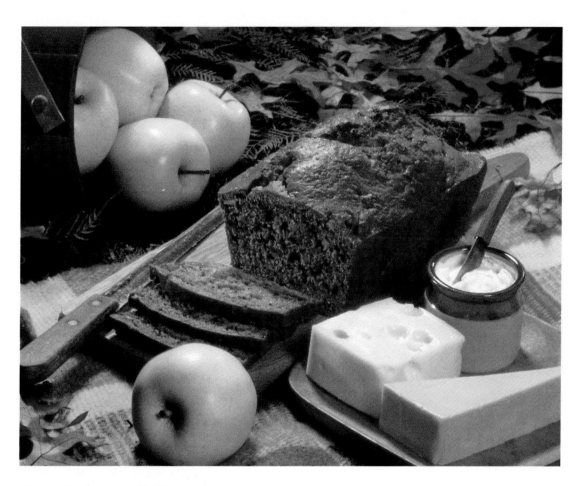

Spicy Applesauce (left)

Golden Apple Wheat Bread

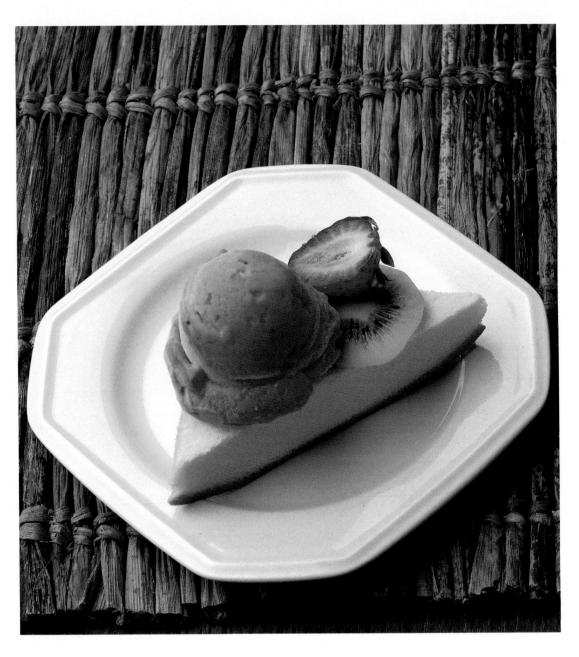

Light and Easy Poundcake

Cranberry Orange Bar Cookies

TWENTY-FOUR COOKIES

1 cup crushed or chopped cranberries
2 oranges, ground with rind
½ cup unsweetened crushed pineapple
1 cup dark or light brown sugar
1⅓ cups liquid margarine
4 eggs
4 teaspoons vanilla extract
8 cups all-purpose flour
4 teaspoons baking powder
2 teaspoons baking soda

Exchange Values
Per Cookie:
2½ Bread
2 Fat

298 Calories
(34% from Fat)
43.1gm Carbohydrates
5.6gm Protein
11.3gm Fat
45.7mg Cholesterol
257mg Sodium
117mg Potassium

Combine all of the ingredients. Press into a 1-inch deep pan. Bake at 350° for 12 to 15 minutes or until firm. Cut into bars while hot. Remove from the pan when cool.

Fruit Cookies

THIRTY-TWO COOKIES

½ cup oil
½ cup dark or light brown sugar
1 egg
1¼ cups all-purpose flour
½ teaspoon baking powder
1 teaspoon cinnamon
¼ teaspoon ground cloves
¼ teaspoon ground allspice
¼ cup skim milk
1 6-ounce package dried mixed fruit bits
1 cup orange juice

Exchange Values
Per Cookie:
½ Fruit
½ Bread
½ Fat

84 Calories
(39% from Fat)
12.1gm Carbohydrates
1gm Protein
3.7gm Fat
8.8mg Cholesterol
10mg Sodium
75mg Potassium

Combine all of the ingredients and mix well. Drop by spoonfuls onto an ungreased cookie sheet. Bake at 350° for 10 to 12 minutes. Cool on a wire rack.

Oat Bran Cookies

THIRTY-TWO COOKIES

½ cup vegetable oil
½ cup dark or light brown sugar
1   egg
2   cups oats
1½ cups oat bran
1   cup all-purpose flour
1   cup applesauce
½ teaspoon baking powder
1   teaspoon ground cinnamon
¼ teaspoon ground cloves
¼ teaspoon ground allspice
¼ cup skim milk
¼ cup orange juice
½ cup chopped walnuts

Exchange Values
Per Cookie:
1 Bread
1 Fat

97 Calories
(45% from Fat)
12.2gm Carbohydrates
1.6gm Protein
5.1gm Fat
8.8mg Cholesterol
24mg Sodium
84mg Potassium

Combine all of the ingredients and mix well. Drop by spoonfuls onto an ungreased cookie sheet and bake at 350° for 10 to 15 minutes.

Peanut Butter Cookies

THIRTY-TWO COOKIES

½ cup liquid margarine
¼ cup sugar
¼ cup creamy peanut butter
¼ cup orange juice
¼ cup water
1 teaspoon vanilla extract
1 egg
2 cups all-purpose flour
2 teaspoons baking powder

Exchange Values
Per Cookie:
½ Bread
1 Fat

75 Calories
(49% from Fat)
8.1gm Carbohydrates
1.6gm Protein
4.1gm Fat
8.6mg Cholesterol
66mg Sodium
29mg Potassium

Combine all of the ingredients in a large bowl. Chill for 2 hours. Roll into balls and place on a cookie sheet. Press down with a fork. Bake at 350° for 10 to 12 minutes.

Oatmeal Cookies

TEN COOKIES

2 cups old-fashioned oats, uncooked
½ cup oat bran cereal
¾ teaspoon baking soda
1 tablespoon cooking oil
½ cup egg substitute
1 teaspoon vanilla extract
1 cup unsweetened crushed pineapple, undrained
1 medium banana, mashed
½ cup raisins
¼ teaspoon cinnamon
⅛ teaspoon nutmeg

Exchange Values
Per Cookie:
½ Fruit
1 Bread
½ Fat

136 Calories
(21% from Fat)
24.1gm Carbohydrates
4.9gm Protein
3.1gm Fat
0mg Cholesterol
108mg Sodium
272mg Potassium

*M*ix all of the ingredients together with a spoon. Form into circles on a sprayed cookie sheet. Bake at 350° for 12 minutes.

Rolled Sugar Cookies

THIRTY-SIX COOKIES

½ cup liquid margarine
½ cup sugar
1 teaspoon vanilla extract
1 egg
2 cups all-purpose flour
½ cup orange juice
2 teaspoons baking powder

Exchange Values
Per Cookie:
½ Bread
½ Fat

62 Calories
(40% from Fat)
8.4gm Carbohydrates
0.9gm Protein
2.7gm Fat
7.6mg Cholesterol
50mg Sodium
17mg Potassium

*C*ream together the margarine, sugar, vanilla, and egg. Add the flour, orange juice, and baking powder until workable and not sticky. Roll on a floured surface and cut into shapes. Place on an ungreased cookie sheet. Bake at 350° until lightly browned.

Russian Tea Cakes

1 cup liquid margarine
¼ cup confectioners' sugar
1 teaspoon vanilla extract
2 cups all-purpose flour
¼ teaspoon cinnamon
½ cup chopped pecans, toasted
¼ cup sugar-free dipping chocolate

*C*ream together the margarine, sugar, and vanilla until light and fluffy. Mix in the flour, cinnamon, and pecans. Roll into ½-inch balls and place on ungreased cookie sheets. Bake at 375° for 15 minutes or until the bottoms brown. Cool on wire rack. When cool, melt the sugar-free dipping chocolate and dip the tops of the cookies in chocolate. Let dry.

Exchange Values
Per Cake:
½ Bread
1 Fat

75 Calories
(66% from Fat)
5.6gm Carbohydrates
0.8gm Protein
5.6gm Fat
0mg Cholesterol
50mg Sodium
19mg Potassium

Peanut Butter Balls

1 .7-ounce box sugar-free white frosting mix
2 tablespoons peanut butter
1 1.3-ounce package sugar-free vanilla pudding
½ cup egg substitute
1 tablespoon margarine
1 tablespoon Galliano liqueur
■ ■ ■
Sugar-free dipping chocolate

*C*ombine all of the ingredients and mix well. The mixture should not be sticky. Roll into balls. Freeze and dip into sugar-free dipping chocolate.

Exchange Values
Per Ball:
½ Fat

25 Calories
(59% from Fat)
1.4gm Carbohydrates
1.2gm Protein
1.7gm Fat
0.7mg Cholesterol
21mg Sodium
17mg Potassium

Diabetic Rum Truffle Candy

EIGHT BALLS

1 .7-ounce box sugar-free white frosting mix
2 tablespoons cocoa
½ cup egg subsitute
1 tablespoon margarine at room temperature
1 tablespoon rum flavoring

*Exchange Values
Per Ball:*
1 Fat

49 Calories
(75% from Fat)
2.6gm Carbohydrates
3.4gm Protein
4.1gm Fat
0mg Cholesterol
56mg Sodium
101mg Potassium

*M*ix all of the ingredients well. The mixture should not be too sticky and needs to be of a consistency to roll into balls.

These can be dipped in sugar-free dipping chocolate but must be frozen before being dipped (not included in analysis).

Apple Gelatin Dessert

TEN SERVINGS

6 3-ounce packages sugar-free strawberry gelatin
5 cups boiling water
3 cups diced apples
2 bananas, diced
1 cup unsweetened crushed pineapple

■ ■ ■

1 packet artificial sweetener
½ cup plain lowfat yogurt
1 cup nondairy whipped topping
⅛ teaspoon cinnamon
½ cup chopped nuts

*Exchange Values
Per Serving:*
1 Bread
1 Fat

135 Calories
(40% from Fat)
16.2gm Carbohydrates
5.3gm Protein
6gm Fat
0.7mg Cholesterol
31mg Sodium
319mg Potassium

*D*issolve the gelatin in the water. Cool until slightly thickened. Add the apples, bananas, and pineapple, and stir until well blended. Pour into a 9x13 pan and chill until firm.

For the topping, whip the sweetener, yogurt and nondairy topping together. Add the cinnamon and blend well. Spoon over the top and sprinkle with chopped nuts.

Crispy Cheesy Apples

SIX SERVINGS

6 cups pared, sliced apples
1 teaspoon cinnamon
½ cup apple cider
■ ■ ■
⅔ cup all-purpose flour
¼ teaspoon salt substitute
½ cup liquid margarine
¼ cup cracker crumbs
1 cup grated lowfat Cheddar cheese

*Exchange Values
Per Serving:*
1½ Fruit
1 Bread
1 Meat
3 Fat

*357 Calories
(46% from Fat)*
41.8gm Carbohydrates
9.4gm Protein
18.1gm Fat
3.9mg Cholesterol
621mg Sodium
271mg Potassium

*A*rrange the apples in a sprayed baking dish. Sprinkle them with cinnamon and pour the cider over. Combine the flour, salt substitute, margarine, cracker crumbs, and cheese. Mix until of the consistency of a streusel. Sprinkle the top of the apples with this mixture. Bake at 350° for 1 hour or until the apples are tender.

Old-Fashioned Apple Crunch

SIX SERVINGS

1 cup oats
½ cup all-purpose flour
1 teaspoon cinnamon
½ cup liquid margarine
■ ■ ■
3 cups chopped apples
1 tablespoon all-purpose flour
1 teaspoon cinnamon
1 tablespoon orange juice
2 packets artificial sweetener

*Exchange Values
Per Serving:*
½ Fruit
1 Bread
3 Fat

*263 Calories
(56% from Fat)*
26.3gm Carbohydrates
3.8gm Protein
16.4gm Fat
0mg Cholesterol
150mg Sodium
147mg Potassium

*M*ix the oats, ½ cup of flour, cinnamon, and margarine until crumbly in texture. Place ½ of the mixture in the bottom of the baking pan. Combine the apples, 1 tablespoon of flour, cinnamon, juice, and sweetener. Spread over the oat mixture. Cover with the remainder of the oat mixture. Bake at 350° for 45 minutes.

Baked Fancy Apples

6 small apples, peeled and cored
½ cup raisins
½ cup orange juice
Grated rind of 1 orange
½ cup pineapple juice

*P*eel and core the apples and place in a baking casserole dish. Fill the center of the apples with the raisins. Mix the orange juice and pineapple juice and spoon over the top of the apples. Sprinkle the apples with the orange rind. Cover and bake at 350° for 30 to 35 minutes.

Exchange Values
Per Serving:
2 Fruit

105 Calories
(3% from Fat)
27.4gm Carbohydrates
0.7gm Protein
0.4gm Fat
0mg Cholesterol
4mg Sodium
254mg Potassium

Blueberry Slump

3 cups blueberries
¼ cup orange juice
1 packet artificial sweetener
½ teaspoon cinnamon

1 cup all-purpose flour
2 teaspoons baking powder
1 tablespoon sugar
½ cup skim milk
3 tablespoons liquid margarine

*S*pray a casserole dish. Place the blueberries in the dish and top with the orange juice. Combine the fructose and cinnamon, and sprinkle over the berries. In a separate bowl combine all of the dry ingredients and make a well in the center. Add the skim milk and begin working by hand. Add the margarine and continue to work by hand. Drop by spoonfuls onto the blueberries. Bake in a 350° oven for 20 minutes or until golden brown. Serve warm.

Exchange Values
Per Serving:
1 Fruit
1 Bread
1 Fat

183 Calories
(30% from Fat)
29.3gm Carbohydrates
3.4gm Protein
6.2gm Fat
0.5mg Cholesterol
172mg Sodium
144mg Potassium

Blueberry Crepes

ONE SERVING

½ cup fresh or frozen blueberries
1 teaspoon vanilla extract
1 packet sugar substitute

■ ■ ■

1 egg white
¼ cup plain lowfat yogurt
1 slice white bread, cubed
Pinch ground cinnamon
½ teaspoon vanilla extract

*Exchange Values
Per Serving:*
1 Fruit
1 Bread
1 Meat

186 Calories
(9% from Fat)
29.6gm Carbohydrates
8.9gm Protein
1.9gm Fat
3.5mg Cholesterol
223mg Sodium
266mg Potassium

Combine the blueberries and vanilla in a saucepan. Barely cover with water and bring to a slow boil over medium heat. Cook uncovered, stirring often, until the consistency of preserves. Remove from the heat, cover, and let cool for five minutes. Add the envelope of sugar substitute.

Combine the egg white, yogurt, bread cubes, cinnamon and vanilla in a blender jar. Blend until smooth. Heat a 10-inch nonstick skillet over low heat and pour in the blender contents, tilting the pan to spread evenly. Lift the edges with rubber spatula, turn only when brown-flecked (or the pancake may tear). Cook the other side. Spread the fruit in the center and roll up.

Crumbly Peaches

SIX SERVINGS

3 cups sliced peaches (fresh work best)
2 cups oat bran
½ cup oat flakes
½ cup whole wheat flour
¼ cup slivered almonds (optional, not in analysis)
2 tablespoons sugar
¼ teaspoon cinnamon
2 tablespoons liquid margarine
1 teaspoon butter-flavored extract

*Exchange Values
Per Serving:*
1 Fruit
1 Bread
1 Fat

*P*lace the peaches in a square casserole. Combine the dry ingredients and then add the margarine and extract. Work by hand until crumbly. Spread over the peaches and bake at 375° for 35 minutes or until golden.

206 Calories
(24% from Fat)
41.4gm Carbohydrates
5.8gm Protein
5.6gm Fat
0mg Cholesterol
190mg Sodium
508mg Potassium

Baked Whole Peaches

FOUR SERVINGS

1 cup all-purpose flour
1 teaspoon salt substitute
¼ cup liquid margarine
3 tablespoons cold sugar-free lemon-lime soda

■ ■ ■

4 whole, unpeeled, perfect peaches

■ ■ ■

2 teaspoons liquid margarine
Cinnamon to sprinkle

Exchange Values
Per Serving:
1 Fruit
1½ Bread
2½ Fat

278 Calories
(44% from Fat)
35.8gm Carbohydrates
4.2gm Protein
13.7gm Fat
0mg Cholesterol
132mg Sodium
290mg Potassium

*M*ix together the flour, salt substitute, and ¼ cup of margarine until of coarse consistency. Add the liquid and mix by hand. Form into 4 balls and roll out similar to a pie crust. Place each peach in the center of a circle of dough just big enough to completely cover the peach. Do not overdo it, just seal the peach completely in a crust. Place on a baking dish and brush the top with margarine. Sprinkle with a small amount of cinnamon. Bake at 400° for 35 to 40 minutes, until golden in color and the crust is flaky. The skin of the peach will disappear when cooked. To serve, open the peach with a knife by cutting down the center. Remove the stone and eat.

Peach and Orange Fluff

EIGHT SERVINGS

2 1.3-ounce packages sugar-free orange gelatin
2 cups boiling water
1½ cups sugar-free orange soda
1 16-ounce can unsweetened sliced peaches, drained
½ cup nondairy whipped topping
½ cup lowfat cottage cheese

*D*issolve the gelatin in 2 cups of boiling water. Allow to thicken, then add the cold sugar-free orange soda. Whip in a blender. Add the peaches, whipped topping, and cottage cheese, and continue to whip until thoroughly combined. Spoon into tall dessert glasses.

Exchange Values
Per Serving:
1 Fruit

47 Calories
(8% from Fat)
5.1gm Carbohydrates
3.5gm Protein
1.3gm Fat
1.2mg Cholesterol
22mg Sodium
99mg Potassium

Peaches 'n' Cream Truffles

EIGHT SERVINGS

1 .7-ounce box sugar-free white frosting mix
1 .3-ounce package vanilla sugar-free pudding mix
½ cup egg substitute
1 tablespoon liquid margarine
1 tablespoon Peach Schnapps

*C*ombine all of the ingredients and mix well. The mixture should not be sticky. Roll into balls. These can be frozen and then dipped in sugar-free white dipping chocolate (not included in analysis).

Exchange Values
Per Truffle:
1 Fat

52 Calories
(71% from Fat)
2.8gm Carbohydrates
1.0gm Protein
4.1gm Fat
0mg Cholesterol
73mg Sodium
18mg Potassium

Pears with Raspberry Sauce

SIX SERVINGS

6 small firm ripe pears
4 cups cold water
¼ cup lemon juice

■ ■ ■

1 cup fresh or frozen unsweetened raspberries
½ cup fresh unsweetened orange juice
2 tablespoons fresh lime juice
3 packets sugar substitute

*Exchange Values
Per Serving:*
1½ Fruit

89 Calories
(6% from Fat)
22.1gm Carbohydrates
0.8gm Protein
0.6gm Fat
0mg Cholesterol
3mg Sodium
225mg Potassium

*P*eel the pears, leaving the stems. Cut a thin slice off the bottom of each so they will stand upright. Place the pears in a large saucepan, and add the cold water and lemon juice. Bring to a boil, reduce the heat and simmer, covered, for 10 to 15 minutes. Drain. Place in a baking dish, cover, and chill for 3 hours or overnight.

For the raspberry sauce, place the raspberries, orange juice, lime juice, and sugar substitute in a blender container. Blend on high speed for 1 minute. Strain to remove the seeds, if desired.

To serve, place the pears in serving dishes and pour the raspberry sauce over the pears.

Strawberry and Orange Pops

SIX SERVINGS

2 cups mashed fresh or frozen strawberries
1 cup fresh or reconstituted frozen unsweetened orange juice
½ cup sugar-free red pop
6 packets artificial sweetener
1 teaspoon fresh lemon or lime juice

*Exchange Values
Per Serving:*
1 Fruit

44 Calories
(6% from Fat)
9.4gm Carbohydrates
0.7gm Protein
0.3gm Fat
0mg Cholesterol
6mg Sodium
200mg Potassium

*B*lend all of the ingredients with a wire whisk or in a food processor. Divide the mixture into six 5-ounce paper cups. Place in a freezer and allow to partially freeze. Place a plastic spoon or popsicle stick in the center of each serving. Freeze solid. To serve, remove from the freezer and allow to warm for a few minutes at room temperature. Tear the paper cup off and enjoy.

Strawberry Parfait

FOUR SERVINGS

1   cup sliced fresh or thawed frozen strawberries, drained
¾ cup boiling water
1   3-ounce package sugar-free strawberry gelatin
½ cup cold sugar-free red pop
    Ice cubes
1   cup thawed nondairy whipped topping
½ teaspoon strawberry flavoring

Exchange Values
Per Serving:
½ Fruit
1 Fat

80 Calories
(55% from Fat)
7.2gm Carbohydrates
1.9gm Protein
4.9gm Fat
0mg Cholesterol
18mg Sodium
107mg Potassium

*S*poon the strawberries into parfait glasses. Pour the boiling water into a blender. Add the gelatin. Cover and blend at low speed until the gelatin is completely dissolved, about 30 seconds. Combine the red pop and ice cubes to make 1¼ cups. Add to the gelatin and stir until the ice is partially melted. Add the whipped topping and strawberry flavoring. Blend at high speed for 30 seconds. Pour over the berries in the glasses. Chill until set, about 30 minutes.

Chocolate Mousse Pudding

FOUR SERVINGS

1½ cups cold skim milk
1   3-ounce package sugar-free instant chocolate pudding
1   cup thawed nondairy whipped topping

Exchange Values
Per Serving:
½ Milk
1 Fat

101 Calories
(44% from Fat)
11gm Carbohydrates
3.4gm Protein
4.9gm Fat
1.5mg Cholesterol
63mg Sodium
156mg Potassium

*P*our the cold skim milk into a bowl. Add the pudding mix and start mixing on a low speed. When it begins to thicken, remove the mixer and use a spoon to fold in the whipped topping. Spoon into wine glasses and garnish with a dollop of whipped topping and a mint leaf.

Cranberry and Pineapple Sherbet

EIGHT SERVINGS

1 3-ounce package sugar-free raspberry gelatin
1 cup boiling low-calorie cranberry juice cocktail
1 cup cold low-calorie cranberry juice cocktail
1 cup crushed unsweetened pineapple
1 cup evaporated skim milk

*D*issolve the gelatin in the boiling cranberry juice. Add the remaining cold juice and beat with an electric beater or wire whisk until well blended. Add the pineapple and milk and mix well. Freeze in a shallow pan until crystals form about 1 inch from the edge of the pan. This takes about 1½ hours. Beat until creamy. Return the mixture to the pan and freeze, stirring occasionally, until the mixture is frozen but slightly mushy—about 1½ to 2 hours.

Exchange Values Per Serving:
1 Fruit

51 Calories
(2% from Fat)
9.2gm Carbohydrates
3gm Protein
0.1gm Fat
1.3mg Cholesterol
69mg Sodium
145mg Potassium

Yogurt Pudding

FOUR SERVINGS

1 1.3-ounce package sugar-free instant vanilla pudding
1 cup skim milk
2 packets artificial sweetener
1 cup plain lowfat yogurt
8 tablespoons nondairy whipped topping

*W*hip the vanilla pudding and milk with a mixer. Add the sweetener and yogurt and spoon into wine glasses. Top each with 2 tablespoons of nondairy whipped topping.

Exchange Values Per Serving:
½ Milk
½ Bread
½ Fat

107 Calories
(28% from Fat)
17.4gm Carbohydrates
5.3gm Protein
3.3gm Fat
4.5mg Cholesterol
146mg Sodium
235mg Potassium

Frozen Banana Yogurt

SIX SERVINGS

1 ¼-ounce envelope unflavored gelatin
¼ cup unsweetened orange juice

■ ■ ■

5 packets sugar substitute
1 cup mashed very ripe bananas
1 tablespoon lemon juice
1 8-ounce container plain lowfat yogurt

■ ■ ■

2 egg whites

Exchange Values Per Serving:
1 Fruit

75 Calories
(10% from Fat)
12.6gm Carbohydrates
4.5gm Protein
0.8gm Fat
2mg Cholesterol
48mg Sodium
271mg Potassium

Sprinkle the gelatin over the orange juice in a small saucepan. Place over low heat and stir constantly until the gelatin dissolves, about 3 minutes. Remove from the heat. Add the sugar substitute and stir. Stir in the bananas and lemon juice. Stir in the yogurt. Pour into a freezer tray or metal loaf pan. Freeze until firm. When frozen solid, break up the frozen mixture in a large bowl and add the egg whites. Beat at high speed with an electric mixer until smooth, about 10 minutes. Return to the pan and freeze. Store in a covered freezer container.

Miscellaneous

Hot Apple Cereal

FOUR SERVINGS

4 **cups skim milk**
2 **teaspoons liquid margarine**
½ **teaspoon cinnamon**
¼ **teaspoon nutmeg**

■ ■ ■

2 **cups rolled oats**
2 **cups peeled, chopped apples**
½ **cup walnuts**
¼ **cup raisins**

■ ■ ■

8 **packets sugar substitute**

Exchange Values
Per Serving:
1 Milk
1 Fruit
2 Bread
3 Fat

422 Calories
(31% from Fat)
57.4gm Carbohydrates
17.4gm Protein
14.4gm Fat
2.7mg Cholesterol
157mg Sodium
763mg Potassium

*C*ombine the milk, margarine, cinnamon, and nutmeg; scald. Add the remaining ingredients except the sugar substitute and place in a sprayed 2-quart casserole. Cover. Bake at 350° for 45 minutes or microwave for 10 minutes at full power. Stir several times, add the sugar substitute, and stir.

Hot Apple Cinnamon Cereal

SIX SERVINGS

4 cups skim milk
½ cup brown sugar
½ teaspoon cinnamon

■ ■ ■

2 cups rolled oats
2 cups peeled and chopped apples
1 cup walnuts (optional, not in analysis)
¼ cup raisins
½ cup wheat germ

*C*ombine the milk, brown sugar, and cinnamon. Scald. Combine with the remaining ingredients in a greased 2-quart casserole. Cover, and bake at 350° for 45 minutes or microwave for 10 minutes at full power. Stir several times.

*Exchange Values
Per Serving:*
1 Milk
1 Fruit
1 Bread
½ Fat

235 Calories
(13% from Fat)
40.1gm Carbohydrates
13.0gm Protein
3.3gm Fat
2.7mg Cholesterol
110mg Sodium
525mg Potassium

Crock Pot Applesauce

NINE SERVINGS

2 pounds Rome Beauty apples (about 9 small)
2 tablespoons lemon juice
1 cup water

■ ■ ■

½ teaspoon cinnamon
1 teaspoon vanilla extract
¼ teaspoon nutmeg
4 packets artificial sweetener

*P*eel and thinly slice the apples. Place in crock pot. Combine the lemon juice and water, and pour over the apples. Cover and cook until the apples are very soft and tender. Pour from the crock pot into a large bowl and with a wooden spoon mix the spices and artificial sweetener to the apples. Pack into jars, cover, and store in the refrigerator. Serve warm or chilled.

*Exchange Values
Per Serving:*
1 Fruit

59 Calories
(5% from Fat)
15.1gm Carbohydrates
0.3gm Protein
0.4gm Fat
0mg Cholesterol
1mg Sodium
93mg Potassium

Applesauce

FOUR SERVINGS

8 **small cooking apples**
1 **cup water**

   ■ ■ ■

1 **teaspoon cinnamon**
½ **teaspoon nutmeg**
4 **packets sugar substitute**

*P*eel, core, and slice the apples. Place in a deep pot. Add the water and bring to a boil. Lower to a simmer and cook until the apples are tender. Mash the apples with a potato masher to a lumpy sauce consistency. Remove from the heat and add the cinnamon, nutmeg, and sugar substitute. Stir well and place in jars. Refrigerate.

Exchange Values
Per Serving:
1 Fruit

67 Calories
(5% from Fat)
16.9gm Carbohydrates
0.2gm Protein
0.4gm Fat
0mg Cholesterol
0mg Sodium
130mg Potassium

Spicy Applesauce

EIGHT SERVINGS

8 **small apples**
⅓ **cup water**
  Strip of lemon or lime peel
1 **2-inch stick cinnamon**
3 **allspice berries**
8 **whole cloves**
2 **packets artificial sweetener**

*C*ore the unpeeled apples and cut into eighths. Add water, lemon peel and spices and simmer about 15 minutes or until soft. Press through a food mill or sieve. Add the sweetener. Chill.

Exchange Values
Per Serving:
1½ Fruit

89 Calories
(4% from Fat)
23.3gm Carbohydrates
0.3gm Protein
0.5gm Fat
0mg Cholesterol
1mg Sodium
162mg Potassium

Cucumber Sauce for Fish, Meats or Vegetables

THIRTY-FIVE SERVINGS

2 cups minced cucumbers, seeds removed
2 teaspoons salt substitute

■ ■ ■

2 cups plain lowfat yogurt
1 cup reduced calorie mayonnaise
1 tablespoon lemon juice or to taste
¼ cup minced onion
¼ cup chopped fresh dill
1 teaspoon sugar
¼ cup chopped fresh parsley
White pepper

Exchange Values
Per 2 Tablespoons:
½ Fat

31 Calories
(67% from Fat)
1.9gm Carbohydrates
0.8gm Protein
2.3gm Fat
3mg Cholesterol
50mg Sodium
155mg Potassium

*P*lace the cucumbers in a large bowl, add the salt substitute, and blend well. Place in a sieve to drain for 20 minutes. Press the cucumbers against the sieve to squeeze out the excess moisture. Place the yogurt in a mixing bowl, stir in the mayonnaise and then the lemon juice. Add the remaining ingredients and mix well. Stir in the cucumbers.

Yogurt and Dill Seafood Sauce

TWENTY TABLESPOONFULS

½ cup plain lowfat yogurt
1 tablespoon lemon juice
1 teaspoon brown mustard
1 tablespoon finely chopped fresh dill
1 tablespoon grated onion
½ cup finely chopped cucumber, well drained

Exchange Values
Per Tablespoon:
Free

5 Calories
(84% from Fat)
0.7gm Carbohydrates
0.4gm Protein
0.1gm Fat
0mg Cholesterol
8mg Sodium
24mg Potassium

*I*n a blender combine all of the ingredients until well blended. Chill. Serve with fish, shrimp or any other wonderful seafood dish. Three tablespoonfuls several times a day is allowed.

Louisiana Creole Barbecue Sauce

THIRTY-TWO TABLESPOONFULS

1 cup finely chopped onion
3 tablespoons safflower oil

■ ■ ■

2 cups tomatoes, skinned
¼ cup white wine vinegar
¼ cup lemon juice
3 tablespoons Worcestershire sauce
1 tablespoon soy sauce
2 tablespoons brown mustard
8 drops Tabasco sauce
1 crushed garlic clove
1 bay leaf
¾ teaspoon chili powder

■ ■ ■

2 tablespoons brown sugar substitute

Exchange Values
Per 3 Tablespoons:
1 Vegetable
1 Fat

77 Calories
(61% from Fat)
6.7gm Carbohydrates
1.4gm Protein
5.6gm Fat
0mg Cholesterol
306mg Sodium
187mg Potassium

*S*auté the onion in the oil until tender. Add the remaining ingredients except the brown sugar substitute and bring to a boil. Reduce the heat to a simmer for 20 minutes. Remove from the heat and allow to cool. When cooled to slightly warm, add the brown sugar substitute and stir well. Serve over beef or chicken. This can be refrigerated and used later.

Maple Syrup

TWELVE TABLESPOONFULS

1¼ cups cold water
1 tablespoon cornstarch
1 teaspoon maple flavoring
10 packets artificial sweetener

Exchange Values
Per Tablespoon:
Free

10 Calories
(0% from Fat)
2.6gm Carbohydrates
0gm Protein
0gm Fat
0mg Cholesterol
11mg Sodium
8mg Potassium

*P*ut the water, cornstarch, and flavoring in a saucepan. Bring to a boil. Remove from the heat and allow to cool. Add the artificial sweetener at this time. Stir well until dissolved. Serve hot or cold over pancakes or waffles. Stir before serving. Two tablespoons several times a day is allowed.

Recipes Index

A Carrot Cocktail, 66
A Fruit Shake, 62
A Fruity Punch, 61
Ale-Poached Fish with Pimiento Sauce, 143
An Apricot Drink, 57
A Peach of a Punch, 53
Appetizers, 37-48
Apples
  Apple-Apricot Pie, 192
  Apple Bread Dressing, 128
  Apple-Cranberry Cobbler, 192
  Apple Gelatin Dessert, 203
  Apple Nut Salad, 80
  Apple-Orange Cider Salad, 80
  Apple-Raisin Muffins, 117
  Apples and Onions Side Dish, 177
  Applesauce, 215
  Applesauce Cake, 189
  Baked Fancy Apples, 205
  Chicken-Apple Dressing, 129
  Christmas Wassail, 50
  Crock Pot Applesauce, 214
  Dutch Apple Pie, 193
  Gingered Fruit Compote, 83
  Golden Apple Wheat Loaf, 116
  Hot Apple Cereal, 213
  Hot Apple Cinnamon Cereal, 214
  Molded Tart Apple Salad, 84
  Old-Fashioned Apple Crunch, 204
  Pumpkin-Apple Bran Muffins, 122
  Pumpkin-Apple Bread, 114
  Skillet Apple Potato Salad, 79
  Spicy Applesauce, 215
  Squash and Apple Dish, 182
  Tropical Fruit Salad, 87
Apricots
  An Apricot Drink, 57

Apple-Apricot Pie, 192
Apricot Chicken, 132
Apricot Cookies, 198
Apricot Oat Bran Muffins, 118
Artichoke Spread, 40
Asparagus and Basil, 169

Baked Beef Tenderloin with Vegetables, 153
Baked Broccoli, 170
Baked Chicken and Rice, 131
Baked Fancy Apples, 205
Baked Fluffy Potatoes, 179
Baked Fried Chicken, 133
Baked Grilled Cheese Sandwich, 130
Baked Italian Onions, 177
Baked Pumpkin Pie, 195
Baked Spicy Shrimp, 150
Baked Whole Peaches, 207
Baked Zucchini and Cheese, 184
Bananas
  Banana Bread, 116
  Banana Muffins, 118
  Blueberry Banana Muffins, 117
  Frozen Banana Yogurt, 212
  Fruity Good Morning Drink, 61
  Gingered Fruit Compote, 83
  Mellow Ambrosia, 84
  Oat Bran-Banana Muffins, 121
  Oatmeal-Banana Muffins, 122
  Tropical Fruit Salad, 87
Bavarian Whipped Strawberry Pie, 197
Beef
  Baked Beef Tenderloin with Vegetables, 153
  Beef and Barley Soup, 91
  Beef and Noodles, 153
  Beef Stew Base, 92
  Chinese Green Pepper Steak, 155

Christmas Night Miniature Meatballs, 42
Fall Apple Pot Roast, 154
Family Beef Stew, 93
Holiday Beef Steaks with Vegetable Sauté and
  Hot Mustard Sauce, 154
Italian Feast, 156
Lentil Bean and Beef Soup, 97
Manicotti with Eggplant-Tomato Relish, 166
Meatball Soup, 98
Microwave Beef Roast and Fennel Parmesan, 158
Old-Fashioned Beef, Macaroni and Tomato
  Casserole, 157
Oriental Beef Kabobs, 40
Our Beef Oriental, 158
Pepper Steak, 160
Poached Beef Tenderloin, 159
Round Steak in Wine Sauce, 160
Swedish Meatballs, 161
Sweet Meatballs, 41
Swiss Steak, 161
Beverages, 49-67
Biscuits
  Whole Wheat and Yogurt Biscuits, 124
  Yogurt Drop Biscuits, 123
Blackberries
  Blackberry and Zucchini Bread, 114
  Blackberry Buzz, 57
Black-Eyed Peas and Wild Rice, 178
Blueberries
  Blueberry Banana Muffins, 117
  Blueberry Crepes, 206
  Blueberry Muffins, 119
  Blueberry Slump, 205
Bran Muffins, Pumpkin-Apple, 122
Bread Pudding with Raisins, 190
Breads, 113-129
Breakfast Tomato Juice, 65
Broccoli
  Baked Broccoli, 170
  Broccoli and Herbs, 170
  Broccoli and Rice Casserole, 171
  Broccoli and Rice Casserole, 171
  Broccoli Casserole, 172
  Broccoli Turkey Casserole, 172
  Cream of Broccoli Soup, 102
  Fresh Broccoli and Cauliflower Salad, 71
  Marinated Vegetables, 42
  Munchy Crunchy Vegetable Dip, 48
  Vegetable and Chicken Outdoor Bake, 140
Broiled Fish Steaks and Herbs, 144
Broiled Stuffed Mushrooms, 44
Broiled Tomatoes, 183
Brunch Punch, 58

Buckwheat and Yogurt Pancakes, 126
Buckwheat Buttermilk Pancakes, 126
Buttermilk Biscuits, 123
Buttermilk, Spiced Lowfat, 68
Buttermilk-Style Dressing, 88

Cabbage, Creole, 173
Cajun Green Beans, 175
Cajun Shrimp and Oyster Soup, 96
Cake
  Applesauce Cake, 189
  Classic Sugar-Free Fruitcake, 190
  Light and Easy Poundcake, 191
Candy, Diabetic Rum Truffle, 203
Cantaloupe
  A Fruit Shake, 62
  Cantaloupe Refresher, 58
  Fruit Combo with an Orange Twist, 82
  Tropical Fruit Salad, 87
  Turkey Salad with Cantaloupe, 72
Carrots
  A Carrot Cocktail, 66
  Carrot and Ginger Soup, 99
  Carrot Cake Muffins, 120
  Cream of Carrot Soup, 102
  Italian Carrot Antipasto, 43
  Marinated Vegetables, 42
  Munchy Crunchy Vegetable Dip, 48
  Sweet Carrots with Dill or Basil, 173
  Vegetable and Chicken Outdoor Bake, 140
  Very Orange Salad, 87
Cauliflower
  Crumbly Cauliflower, 174
  Fresh Broccoli and Cauliflower Salad, 71
  Marinated Vegetables, 42
  Vegetable and Chicken Outdoor Bake, 140
Celery Cole Slaw, 70
Cereal
  Hot Apple Cereal, 213
  Hot Apple Cinnamon Cereal, 214
Cheese
  Baked Broccoli, 170
  Baked Grilled Cheese Sandwich, 130
  Baked Zucchini and Cheese, 184
  Broccoli and Rice Casserole, 171
  Broccoli Casserole, 172
  Cheddar Dijon Dip, 45
  Cheese and Sesame Chicken, 132
  Cheesy Scalloped Cucumbers, 174
  Cheesy Scalloped Potatoes, 181
  Cheesy Whipped Potatoes, 179
  Cherry Supreme Cheesecake, 194
  Creole Cabbage, 173

Crispy Cheesy Apples, 204
Crumbly Cauliflower, 174
Lasagna Casserole, 156
Mostaccioli al Forno, 162
Old-Fashioned Macaroni and Cheese, 187
Piney Cheese Ball, 39
Shrimp and Cheese Spread, 39
Spinach-Parmesan Lasagna, 165
Summer Squash Casserole, 181
Vegetarian Lasagna, 164
White Wine Melon and Cheese Appetizer, 38
Vegetarian Lasagna, 164
Zucchini Bake, 185
Zucchini-Ricotta Casserole, 186
Cherry Supreme Cheesecake, 194
Chicken
    Apricot Chicken, 132
    Baked Chicken and Rice, 131
    Baked Fried Chicken, 133
    Cheese and Sesame Chicken, 132
    Chicken-Apple Dressing, 129
    Chicken a l'Orange, 133
    Chicken and Vegetable Soup, 92
    Chicken Popovers, 134
    Chicken Rosemary, 134
    Chicken Salad, 70
    Chicken Tarragon, 135
    Chicken Teriyaki, 135
    Citrus Broiled Chicken, 136
    Cream of Chicken and Wild Rice Soup, 101
    Gingered Lime Chicken, 136
    Gingered Parsnip and Chicken Soup, 94
    Herbed Chicken, 137
    Hot Hot Gumbo, 95
    Kiwi Chicken, 140
    Oven-Baked Chicken Liver, 141
    Poultry and Rice Pilaf, 138
    Roasted Orange Chicken, 138
    Savory Jumbo Shells, 163
    Stir Fry Chicken, 139
    Stuffed Chicken Breasts, 141
    Vegetable and Chicken Outdoor Bake, 140
    Zesty Chicken Italiano, 142
Chili, Family Style, 110
Chinese Green Pepper Steak, 155
Chocolate
    Chocolate Cafe Borgia, 50
    Chocolate-Coffee Milkshake, 53
    Chocolate Mousse Pudding, 210
Chopped Liver, Holiday, 41
Chowders
    Clam Chowder, 109
    Fall Harvest Chowder, 108

Tuna Chowder, 107
    Turkey Chowder, 108
Christmas Night Miniature Meatballs, 42
Christmas Salad, 81
Christmas Wassail, 50
Cinnamon French Toast, 124
Citrus Broiled Chicken, 136
Citrus Punch, 59
Clam Chowder, 109
Classic Sugar-Free Fruitcake, 190
Cobbler, Apple-Cranberry, 192
Coffee
    Chocolate Cafe Borgia, 50
    Chocolate-Coffee Milkshake, 53
    Hot Spiced Coffee, 51
Cold Weather Soup, 98
Cole Slaw, Celery, 70
Colonial Orange Spiced Walnuts, 37
Cookies
    Apricot Cookies, 198
    Cranberry Orange Bar Cookies, 199
    Fruit Cookies, 199
    Oat Bran Cookies, 200
    Peanut Butter Cookies, 200
    Rolled Sugar Cookies, 201
    Russian Tea Cakes, 202
Corn Bread Stuffing, Southern, 129
Corncakes, Old-Fashioned, 127
Cornflake-Breaded Baked Fish, 144
Cornmeal Griddle Pancakes, 127
Cottage Cheese Ranch Dressing, 89
Crab
    Crab Imperial, 148
    Spicy Crab Soup, 94
Crackers, Your Own Crispy, 43
Cranberries
    Apple-Cranberry Cobbler, 192
    Christmas Salad, 81
    Cranberry and Pineapple Sherbet, 211
    Cranberry Fizz Punch, 59
    Cranberry Orange Bar Cookies, 199
    Cranberry-Orange Muffins, 120
    Zesty Cranberry Salad, 88
Creamed Iced Tea, 54
Cream of Broccoli Soup, 102
Cream of Carrot Soup, 102
Cream of Chicken and Wild Rice Soup, 101
Creamy Cucumber Soup, 103
Creole Cabbage, 173
Crispy Cheesy Apples, 204
Crock Pot Applesauce, 214
Crumbly Cauliflower, 174
Crumbly Peaches, 206

Cucumbers
  Cheesy Scalloped Cucumbers, 174
  Creamy Cucumber Soup, 103
  Cucumber Sauce for Fish, Meats, or Vegetables, 216
  Molded Cucumber Salad, 75

Desserts, 189-212
Diabetic Rum Truffle Candy, 203
Dilly Dip, 46
Dips
  Cheddar Dijon Dip, 45
  Dilly Dip, 46
  Guacamole Dip, 46
  Hotty Totty Onion Dip, 47
  Mexican Salsa, 47
  Munchy Crunchy Vegetable Dip, 48
  Spinach Vegetable Dip, 48
Dressings
  Apple Bread Dressing, 128
  Chicken-Apple Dressing, 129
  Mushroom Dressing, 128
Dutch Apple Pie, 193
Dutch Peach Pie, 194

Eggplant
  Eggplant Salad, 69
  Stuffed Eggplant, 175
Entrees, 131-168

Fall Apple Pot Roast, 155
Fall Harvest Chowder, 108
Fall Harvest Soup, 104
Family Beef Stew, 93
Family Style Chili, 110
Fish
  Ale-Poached Fish with Pimiento Sauce, 143
  Broiled Fish Steaks and Herbs, 144
  Cornflake-Breaded Baked Fish, 144
  Fish Almondine, 145
  Flounder Bake, 145
  Seaman's Fish Bake, 149
  Trout Bake, 148
Fluffy Orange Yogurt Salad, 81
French Green Bean and Rice Casserole, 176
French Green Beans Almondine, 176
French Onion Soup "In a Hurry," 99
French Toast, Cinnamon, 124
Fresh Broccoli and Cauliflower Salad, 71
Frosty Strawberry Delight, 60
Frozen Banana Yogurt, 212
Fruit and Nut Curried Salad, 82
Fruit Combo with an Orange Twist, 82

Fruit Cookies, 199
Fruit Cubes and Fizz, 60
Fruity Good Morning Drink, 61
Fruity Slush, 62
Fruity Sweet Potatoes, 180

Garlic and Parmesan Pecans, 38
Gazpacho Salad, 76
Gingered Fruit Compote, 83
Gingered Lime Chicken, 136
Gingered Parsnip and Chicken Soup, 94
Gingered Pineapple Mold, 83
Golden Apple Wheat Loaf, 116
Golden Mediterranean Pilaf, 187
Graham Cracker Crust, 197
Green Beans
  Cajun Green Beans, 175
  French Green Beans Almondine, 176
  French Green Beans and Rice Casserole, 176
  Green Bean Salad, 72
Guacamole Dip, 46
Gumbo, Hot Hot, 95

Hearty Fruit Soup, 110
Hearty Potato Soup, 105
Hearty Tomato Saucy Drink, 67
Herbed Chicken, 137
Herbed Spice Dressing, 89
Holiday Beef Steaks with Vegetable Sauté and Hot Mustard Sauce, 154
Holiday Chopped Liver, 41
Hot Apple Cereal, 213
Hot Apple Cinnamon Cereal, 214
Hot Hot Gumbo, 95
Hot Spiced Coffee, 51
Hot Spiced Tea, 49
Hot Tuna and Potato Bake, 146
Hotty Totty Onion Dip, 47
House Salad with Dream Pepper Dressing, 73

Instant Breakfast Drink, 52
Italian Carrot Antipasto, 43
Italian Feast, 156

Kiwi Chicken, 140

Lasagna Casserole, 156
Leek and Mussel Poach, 152
Lentil Bean and Beef Soup, 97
Lettuce-Baked Lobster Tails, 149
Light and Easy Pound Cake, 191
Lime and Raspberry Refresher, 63

Liver, Holiday Chopped, 41
Lobster Tails, Lettuce Baked, 149
Louisiana Creole Barbecue Sauce, 217

Macaroni and Cheese, Old-Fashioned, 187
Macaroni Salad, 77
Manicotti with Eggplant-Tomato Relish, 166
Manicotti with Ratatouille Sauce, 167
Maple Syrup, 217
Marinated Vegetables, 42
Meatballs
   Christmas Night Miniature Meatballs, 42
   Meatball Soup, 98
   Swedish Meatballs, 161
   Sweet Meatballs, 41
Mellow Ambrosia, 84
Mexican Cherry Tomatoes, 183
Mexican Salsa, 47
Microwave Beef Roast and Fennel Parmesan, 158
Milk, Warmed Wintery, 54
Mint Juleps, Southern, 56
Mint Tea, 56
Miscellaneous, 213-217
Molded Cucumber Salad, 75
Molded Tart Apple Salad, 84
Mostaccioli al Forno, 162
Muffins
   Apple-Raisin Muffins, 117
   Apricot Oat Bran Muffins, 118
   Banana Muffins, 118
   Blueberry Muffins, 119
   Carrot Cake Muffins, 120
   Cranberry-Orange Muffins, 120
   Oat Bran-Banana Muffins, 121
   Oatmeal-Banana Muffins, 122
   Pumpkin-Apple Bran Muffins, 122
Munchy Crunchy Vegetable Dip, 48
Mushrooms
   Broiled Stuffed Mushrooms, 44
   Mushroom Dressing, 128
   Shrimp and Mushrooms, 151
   Stuffed Dill Mushrooms, 44

Oat Bran
   Apricot Oat Bran Muffins, 118
   Oat Bran-Banana Muffins, 121
   Oat Bran Bread, 115
   Oat Bran Cookies, 200
   Oat Bran Muffins, 121
   Oat Bran Pie Crust, 198
   Scottish Oat Bran Toast, 125
Oats
   Oatmeal-Banana Muffins, 122

Oatmeal Cookies, 201
Oriental Oat Pilaf, 186
Scottish Oat Cakes, 125
Your Own Crispy Crackers, 43
Old-Fashioned Apple Crunch, 204
Old-Fashioned Beef, Macaroni and Tomato
   Casserole, 157
Old-Fashioned Corncakes, 127
Old-Fashioned Macaroni and Cheese, 187
Old-Fashioned Potato Salad, 74
Onions
   Apples and Onions Side Dish, 177
   Baked Italian Onions, 177
   French Onion Soup "In a Hurry," 99
   Hotty Totty Onion Dip, 47
   Spaghetti Squash and Vegetables, 182
Oranges
   Apple-Orange Cider Salad, 80
   Citrus Punch, 59
   Colonial Orange Spiced Walnuts, 37
   Cranberry Orange Bar Cookies, 199
   Cranberry-Orange Muffins, 120
   Fluffy Orange Yogurt Salad, 81
   Fruit and Nut Curried Salad, 82
   Fruit Combo with an Orange Twist, 82
   Fruity Good Morning Drink, 61
   Fruity Slush, 62
   Gingered Fruit Compote, 83
   Instant Breakfast Drink, 52
   Mellow Ambrosia, 84
   Orange Curried Rice and Mushrooms, 188
   Orange Frosty, 63
   Orange Monster Drink, 52
   Orange Pineapple Salad, 85
   Peach and Orange Fluff, 208
   Pudding Salad, 86
   Strawberry and Orange Pops, 209
   Tea Punch, 53
   Very Orange Salad, 87
Oriental Beef Kabobs, 40
Oriental Oat Pilaf, 186
Our Beef Oriental, 158
Oven-Baked Chicken Liver, 141
Oysters
   Cajun Shrimp and Oyster Soup, 96
   Oyster Stew, 93
   Rock Shrimp and Oyster Manquechou, 150

Pancakes
   Buckwheat and Yogurt Pancakes, 126
   Buckwheat Buttermilk Pancakes, 126
   Cornmeal Griddle Cakes, 127
   Old-Fashioned Corncakes, 127

Papaya
  A Fruit Shake, 62
  Tropical Fruit Salad, 87
Parmesan Linguine with Garlic, 162
Pasta
  Beef and Noodles, 153
  Gazpacho Salad, 76
  Italian Feast, 156
  Lasagna Casserole, 156
  Macaroni Salad, 77
  Manicotti with Eggplant-Tomato Relish, 166
  Manicotti with Ratatouille Sauce, 167
  Mostaccioli al Forno, 162
  Old-Fashioned Beef, Macaroni and Tomato
    Casserole, 157
  Old-Fashioned Macaroni and Cheese, 187
  Parmesan Linguini with Garlic, 162
  Pasta and Vegetable Salad, 78
  Pasta Salad, 76
  Red Pepper and Pasta Salad, 79
  Savory Jumbo Shells, 163
  Spicy Manicotti, 168
  Spinach-Parmesan Lasagna, 165
  Tuna and Noodle Casserole Bake, 146
  Vegetable and Pasta Soup, 100
Peaches
  A Peach of a Punch, 53
  Baked Whole Peaches, 207
  Crumbly Peaches, 206
  Hearty Fruit Soup, 110
  Peach and Orange Fluff, 208
  Peaches and Cream Salad, 85
  Peaches 'N' Cream Truffles, 208
  Pineapple and Peach Soup, 111
Peanut Butter Balls, 202
Peanut Butter Cookies, 200
Pears with Raspberry Sauce, 209
Pecans, Garlic and Parmesan, 38
Peppers, Stuffed, 178
Pepper Steak, 160
Pie Crusts
  Graham Cracker Crust, 197
  Oat Bran Pie Crust, 198
Pies
  Apple-Apricot Pie, 192
  Bavarian Whipped Strawberry Pie, 197
  Dutch Apple Pie, 193
  Dutch Peach Pie, 194
  Pumpkin Pie in a Graham Cracker Crust, 196
Pineapple
  A Fruity Punch, 61
  Christmas Salad, 81
  Fruit Combo with an Orange Twist, 82

Gingered Pineapple Mold, 83
  Hearty Fruit Soup, 110
  Orange Pineapple Salad, 85
  Pineapple and Peach Soup, 111
  Pudding Salad, 86
  Tart and Bubbly Wake-Up Drink, 65
  Tropical Fruit Salad, 87
  Zesty Cranberry Salad, 88
Piney Cheese Ball, 39
Poached Beef Tenderloin, 159
Potatoes
  Baked Fluffy Potatoes, 179
  Cheesy Scalloped Potatoes, 181
  Cheesy Whipped Potatoes, 179
  Fruity Sweet Potatoes, 180
  Hearty Potato Soup, 105
  Hot Tuna and Potato Bake, 146
  Old-Fashioned Potato Salad, 74
  Potato Leek Soup, 105
  Skillet Apple Potato Salad, 74
  Stuffed Baked Potatoes, 180
  Tuna Potato Casserole, 147
Pot Roast, Fall Apple, 155
Poultry, and Rice Pilaf, 138
Poultry, *see* Chicken, Turkey
Puddings
  Bread Pudding with Raisins, 190
  Chocolate Mousse Pudding, 210
  Yogurt Pudding, 211
Pudding Salad, 86
Pumpkin
  Baked Pumpkin Pie, 195
  Pumpkin-Apple Bran Muffins, 122
  Pumpkin-Apple Bread, 114
  Pumpkin Pie in a Graham Cracker Crust, 196

Red Pepper and Pasta Salad, 79
Refreshing Chilled Strawberry Soup, 112
Rice
  Baked Chicken and Rice, 131
  Black-Eyed Peas and Wild Rice, 178
  Broccoli and Rice Casserole, 171
  Broccoli and Rice Casserole, 171
  Cream of Chicken and Wild Rice Soup, 101
  French Green Bean and Rice Casserole, 176
  Golden Mediterranean Pilaf, 187
  Hot Hot Gumbo, 95
  Orange Curried Rice and Mushrooms, 188
  Poultry and Rice Pilaf, 138
  Wild Rice Salad, 78
Roasted Orange Chicken, 138
Rock Shrimp and Oyster Manquechou, 150
Rolled Sugar Cookies, 201

Round Steak in Wine Sauce, 160
Rum Truffle Candy, Diabetic, 203
Russian Tea Cakes, 202

Salad Dressings
    Cottage Cheese Ranch Dressing, 89
    Herbed Spice Dressing, 89
    Tartar Sauce Dressing, 90
Salads, 69-90
Salsa, Mexican, 47
Sandwich, Baked Grilled Cheese, 130
Sauces
    Cucumber Sauce for Fish, Meats or Vegetables,
        216
    Louisiana Creole Barbecue Sauce, 217
    Yogurt and Dill Seafood Sauce, 216
Savory Jumbo Shells, 163
Savory Zucchini Soup, 104
Scottish Oat-Bran Toast, 125
Scottish Oat Cakes, 125
Seaman's Fish Bake, 149

Shrimp
    Baked Spicy Shrimp, 150
    Cajun Shrimp and Oyster Soup, 96
    Rock Shrimp and Oyster Manquechou, 150
    Shrimp and Cheese Spread, 39
    Shrimp and Mushrooms, 151
Skillet Apple Potato Salad, 74
Soups, 91-112
Southern Corn Bread Stuffing, 129
Southern Mint Julips, 56
Spaghetti Squash and Vegetables, 182
Spiced Lowfat Buttermilk, 68
Spiced Russian Tea, 53
Spicy Applesauce, 215
Spicy Crab Soup, 94
Spicy Manicotti, 168
Spinach
    Mostaccioli al Forno, 162
    Savory Jumbo Shells, 163
    Spinach-Parmesan Lasagna, 165
    Spinach Salad, 75
    Spinach Vegetable Dip, 48
    Vegetarian Lasagna, 164
Squash
    Squash and Apple Dish, 182
    Summer Squash Casserole, 181
Steamed Vegetables, 184
Stew
    Beef Stew Base, 92
    Family Beef Stew, 93
    Oyster Stew, 93

Stir Fry Chicken, 139
Strawberries
    A Fruit Shake, 62
    Bavarian Whipped Strawberry Pie, 197
    Frosty Strawberry Delight, 60
    Fruit Combo with an Orange Twist, 82
    Fruity Good Morning Drink, 61
    Refreshing Chilled Strawberry Soup, 112
    Strawberry and Orange Pops, 209
    Strawberry Gelatin Salad, 86
    Strawberry Grog, 64
    Strawberry Parfait, 210
    Strawberry Parfait Drink, 64
    Summer Strawberry and Burgundy Soup, 112
    Tropical Fruit Salad, 87
Streusel Topping, 196
Stuffed Baked Potatoes, 180
Stuffed Chicken Breasts, 141
Stuffed Dill Mushrooms, 44
Stuffed Eggplant, 175
Stuffed Peppers, 178
Stuffing, Southern Corn Bread, 129
Sweet Potatoes, Fruity, 180
Syrup, Maple, 217
Summer Squash Casserole, 181
Summer Strawberry and Burgundy Soup, 112
Swedish Meatballs, 161
Sweet Carrots with Dill or Basil, 173
Sweet Meatballs, 41
Swiss Steak, 161

Tangy Tomato Aspic, 77
Tart and Bubbly Wake-Up Drink, 65
Tartar Sauce Dressing, 90
Tea
    Citrus Punch, 59
    Creamed Iced Tea, 54
    Hot Spiced Tea, 49
    Instant Breakfast Drink, 52
    Spiced Russian Tea, 53
    Tea Punch, 53
Tea Cakes, Russian, 202
Tofu Soup, 106
Tomatoes
    Breakfast Tomato Juice, 65
    Broiled Tomatoes, 183
    Hearty Tomato Saucy Drink, 67
    Mexican Cherry Tomatoes, 183
    Mexican Salsa, 47
    Spaghetti Squash and Vegetables, 182
    Tangy Tomato Aspic, 77
    Tomato and Celery Curry Drink, 66
    Tomato Frappe, 67

Tropical Fruit Salad, 87
Trout Bake, 148
Truffles, Peaches 'N' Cream, 208
Tuna
   Hot Tuna and Potato Bake, 146
   Tuna and Noodle Casserole Bake, 146
   Tuna Chowder, 107
   Tuna Potato Casserole, 147
   Tuna Salad, 71
Turkey
   Broccoli Turkey Casserole, 172
   Savory Jumbo Shells, 163
   Turkey Chowder, 108
   Turkey Salad with Cantaloupe, 72
   Turkey with Cranberry-Apple Sauce, 142

Veal Provencale, 164
Vegetable and Chicken Outdoor Bake, 140
Vegetable and Pasta Soup, 100
Vegetables and Rice, 169-188
Vegetable Soup, 100
Vegetarian Lasagna, 164
Very Orange Salad, 87

Walnuts, Colonial Orange Spiced, 37
Warmed Wintery Milk, 54

White Wine Melon and Cheese Appetizer, 38
Whole Wheat and Yogurt Biscuits, 124
Whole Wheat Bread, 113
Wild Rice Salad, 78

Yogurt
   Buckwheat and Yogurt Pancakes, 126
   Fluffy Orange Yogurt Salad, 81
   Frozen Banana Yogurt, 212
   Whole Wheat and Yogurt Biscuits, 124
   Yogurt and Dill Seafood Sauce, 216
   Yogurt Drop Biscuits, 123
   Yogurt Pudding, 211
Your Own Crispy Crackers, 43

Zesty Chicken Italiano, 142
Zesty Cranberry Salad, 88
Zucchini
   Baked Zucchini and Cheese, 184
   Blackberry and Zucchini Bread, 114
   Parmesan Linguini with Garlic, 162
   Savory Zucchini Soup, 104
   Zucchini Bake, 185
   Zucchini Casserole, 185
   Zucchini-Ricotta Casserole, 186
   Zucchini Soup, 106

Menu Planning Index

adjustments for travel, 13-14
aerobic exercise, 5
airplane travel, 13
alcohol, 6
American Diabetes Association, 4, 8, 15, 18, 22
American Diabetes Association diet, 2
American Dietetic Association, 4, 22
American Indians, 1
angel food cake, 34
appetite, 2
aspartame, 8, 17, 35

beans, 33
beef, 25, 26, 27
beer, 6
blood lipids, 2, 6
blood sugar, 2, 3, 5, 6, 10, 13, 22
bratwurst, 27
bread, 23, 24
"brittle" Type I diabetes, 2
butterfat, 30

cake, no icing, 34
calcium, 30
caloric sweeteners, 7-8, 17
calories, 23, 25, 30
calories, daily intake, 4
carbohydrates, 13, 22, 23, 25, 30, 34
car travel, lengthy, 13
casseroles, homemade, 33
cereal, 23, 24
cheese, 26, 27

cheese pizza, 33
chicken, 1, 35
children, diabetic, 14-16
chili, 33
cholesterol, 1, 2, 3, 6, 25
cholesterol-lowering diet, 6
chow mein, 33
Chronic Disease Program, 22
"civilized" eating patterns, 1
Combination Foods, 33
condiments, free, 32
cooked foods, 35
cooked vegetables, 28
cookies, 34
Cooper, Dr. Kenneth, 5
corn syrup, 8
coronary artery disease, 2
crackers/snacks, 24
Cream of Wheat, 35

daily caloric needs, 3
dairy products, 1
"diabetic diet," 3
Diabetic Exchange Lists, 23-35
diet, American Diabetes Association, 2
diet and exercise, 1
dietetic, 34
dietician, 3, 6
dried beans, 24, 35
dried fruit, 29
dried peas, 35
drinks, free, 32

eating out, 11-12
eating preferences, 10
eggs, 1, 27
egg substitutes, 26, 27
egg whites, 26
emergency treatment, travel, 14
Equal, 8, 17
Eskimos, 1
exchange lists, 4, 23-35
exercise, 1, 3, 5, 6

fast food, 11
fat, 23, 25, 30
Fat Exchanges, 31
fatty meats, 1
Featherweight, 8
fiber, 6, 23
fiber, sources of, 6
fish, 1, 26, 27
Foods for Occasional Use, 34
frankfurters, 27
Free Foods, 31-33
fresh fruit, 29
frozen fruit yogurt, 34
fructose, 7, 17, 35
fruit, 7
Fruit Exchanges, 29-30
fruit, free, 32
fruit juice, 30

gingersnaps, 34
glucose, 5, 7
glycogen, 7
grain, 23, 24
grits, 35
granola, 34
granola bars, 34

hamburger, 35
hard liquor, 6
heart disease, 1
heart (meat exchanges), 27
heart rate, exercise, 5
high blood pressure, 3
high-fat dairy products, 1
High-Fat Meat and Substitutes, 27
high-fat meat nutrients, 25
high-fiber diet, 6
honey, 7, 8
hypertension, 3
hypoglycemia, 5
hypoglycemic therapy, 3

ice cream, any flavor, 34
ice milk, any flavor, 34

ideal weight, 3
insulin, 2, 3, 6, 13
insulin shock, 5
insulin therapy, 2
insulin, use on airplanes, 13

juvenile-onset diabetes, 2

kidney (meat exchanges), 27
kidney problems, 3
knockwurst, 27

labels, nutritional information on, 17, 34
lamb, 26, 27
Lean Mean and Substitutes, 25
lean meat nutrients, 25
lentils, 24, 35
lipids, blood, 2
liquor, 6
liver (meat exchanges), 27
low blood sugar, 2
low blood sugar reactions, 3
low cholesterol/lowfat diet, 6
lowfat dairy products, 1
lowfat milk, 30
lowfat milk nutrients, 30
luncheon meat, 26, 27

macaroni, 35
macaroni and cheese, 33
Management Tips, 34-35
mannitol, 7, 35
Marshall Plan, 1
maturity-onset diabetes, 2
meals, scheduled, 2, 12
Meat Exchanges, 25-28
meats, fatty, 1
meats group, 35
Medium-Fat Meat and Substitutes, 26
medium-fat meat nutrients, 25
menu, 36
metabolism, 2
Milk Exchanges, 30
minerals, 28

New Aerobic Way, The, 5
new onset of diabetes, 1
non-caloric sugar substitutes, 17-18
nonstick pan spray, 32
non-sugar sweeteners, 8
noodles, 35
Nutra Sweet, 17
nutritional information on labels, 17
nuts and seeds, 31

oatmeal, 35
obesity, 1, 4
oil, 31
1,000 Calorie Daily Food Allowances, 18
1,800 Calorie Daily Food Allowances, 20
1,500 Calorie Daily Food Allowances, 19
1,200 Calorie Daily Food Allowances, 19
oral hypoglycemic agent, 3, 6

pasta, 23, 24
peanut butter, 27
peas, 24
pork, 25, 26, 27
positive attitude, 11
positive family history, 2
poultry, 26
prescribed snacks, 2
protein, 3, 23, 25, 30

raw vegetables, 28
renal disease, 3
restaurants, 11-12
rice, 35
rules and guidelines for exchange lists, 23

saccharin, 8, 17, 35
salad dressing, 31
salad greens, free, 32
Sample 2,000 Calorie Diet Menu, 36
saturated fats, 1, 6, 25, 31
sausage, 27
schedules, 13
seasonings, 32
serving sizes, 35
sherbet, any flavor, 34
skim and very lowfat milk, 30
skim/very lowfat milk nutrients, 30
snack chips, 34
snacks, for travel, 13
snacks, prescribed, 2
snacks, timing of, 3
sodium, 23, 25
sodium-free spices, 3
sodium restriction, 3
Sorbitol, 7, 17, 35
soup, 33
spaghetti, 35
spaghetti and meatballs, 33
Starch-Bread Exchanges, 23-25
starches group, 35
starch foods prepared with fat, 24
starchy vegetables, 24
stress, 10-11

sucrose, 7
sugar, 5-6
sugar-free pudding, 33
Sugars, 7-8
sugar substitutes, 7-8, 17
summer camp for children, 15
support groups, 15
sweetbreads, 27
sweeteners, 7-8, 35
Sweet 'N Low, 8
sweet substitutes, free, 32
syrups, 8

thirst, 2
3,000 Calorie Daily Food Allowances, 21-22
"time out," 11
time zones, 14
timing of regular meals, 3
tofu, 27
travel, 13-14
turkey, 1
2,000 Calorie Daily Food Allowances, 20
2,500 Calorie Daily Food Allowances, 21
Type I diabetes, 2
Type II diabetes, 2

uncooked foods, 35
United States Public Health Service, 4, 22
unsaturated fats, 6, 31
unsweetened canned fruit, 29
urination, frequent, 2

vanilla wafers, 34
veal, 26
Vegetable Exchanges, 28
vegetables, free, 32
vitamins, 28

water, 14
water insoluble fiber, 6
water soluble fiber, 6
weight, adult, 4
weight, ideal, 3-4
weight loss, 6
weight (obesity), 1
whole milk, 30
whole milk nutrients, 30
wild game, 26
wine, 6
World War II, 1

Xylitol, 17